Trigger Point Therapy

for Shoulder Pain

including Frozen Shoulder

(Second Edition)

Valerie DeLaune, LAc

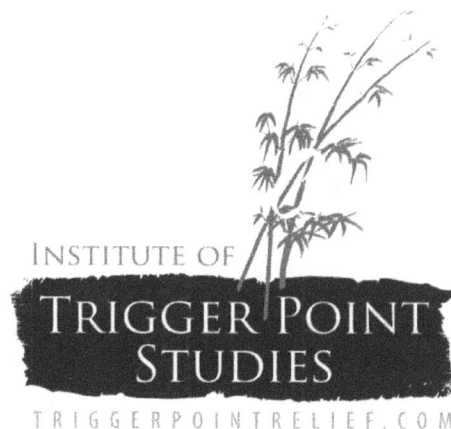

INSTITUTE OF
TRIGGER POINT
STUDIES

TRIGGERPOINTRELIEF.COM

ISBN 13: 978-0-9968553-1-0

First Edition, 2012
Second Edition, 2013

Disclaimer:

The following information is intended for general information purposes only. Individuals should always see their health care provider before administering any suggestions made in this book. Any application of the material set forth in the following pages is at the reader's discretion and is his or her sole responsibility.

This book is intended as a quick-reference only for the major muscles that may harbor trigger points that refer pain to the shoulder area. It is not intended as a comprehensive therapy guide for other areas of the body. If you are unable to relieve all of your pain with the techniques found in this book, you may wish to consult one of the resources found at the end of this book in order to treat other pertinent muscles.

Table of Contents

Acknowledgements

This book would not have been possible without the lifeworks of Dr. Janet Travell and Dr. David G. Simons, who worked endlessly to research trigger points, document referral patterns and other symptoms, and bring all of that information to medical practitioners and the general public. Together Doctors Travell and Simons produced a comprehensive two-volume text on the causes and treatment of trigger points, written for physicians. This text is a condensation of those volumes, written for the general public, and for practitioners who don't need the in-depth knowledge to perform trigger point injections.

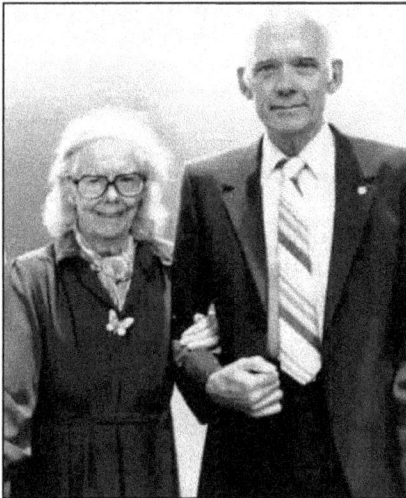

Dr. Janet Travell and Dr. David G. Simons

Dr. Travell pioneered and researched new pain treatments, including trigger point injections. In her private practice, she began treating Senator John F. Kennedy, who at the time was using crutches due to crippling back pain and was almost unable to walk down just a few stairs. It had become important for presidential candidates to appear physically fit, because of television. Being on crutches probably would have cost President Kennedy the election. Dr. Travell became the first female White House physician, and after President Kennedy died, she stayed on to treat President Johnson. She resigned a year and a half later to return to her passions: teaching, lecturing, and writing about chronic myofascial pain. She continued to work into her nineties and died at the age of ninety-five on August 1, 1997.

Dr. Simons met Dr. Travell when she lectured at the School of Aerospace Medicine at Brooks Air Force Base in Texas in the 1960s. He soon teamed up with Dr. Travell and began researching the international literature for any references to the treatment of pain. There were a few others out there who were also discovering trigger points but using different terminology. He studied and documented the physiology of trigger points in both laboratory and clinical settings and tried to find scientific explanations for trigger points. He continued to research the physiology of trigger points, update the trigger point volumes he coauthored with Dr. Travell, and review trigger point research articles until his death at the age of 88 on April 5, 2010.

I am also profoundly grateful to my neuromuscular therapy instructor, Jeanne Aland, who taught me basics about trigger points, and introduced me to the books written by Doctors Travell and Simons. I was told Jeanne passed on a few years ago.

All three are well-missed. Those familiar with trigger points are extremely grateful for their hard work and dedication. Their work lives on through the hundreds of thousands of patients who have gotten relief because of their research and willingness to train others.

Other Thanks

Many additional researchers have contributed to the study of trigger points, and many doctors and other practitioners have taken the time to learn about trigger points and give that information to their patients. I would like to acknowledge all of them for their role in alleviating pain by making this important information available. In particular I would like to thank Dr. Juhani Partanen, who kindly explained the "Muscle Spindle" hypothesis to me in lay terms, and also took the time to review the chapter "Appendix B: What Are Trigger Points?" to make sure I had translated scientific language correctly into easier-to-understand terms.

My Background

I attended massage school in 1989 and learned Swedish massage. I learned to give a very good general massage, but I didn't feel equipped to treat chronic pain. I was very intrigued by a description of a continuing education certificate course; it was called *neuromuscular therapy,* which combines *myofascial release* (a type of deep tissue massage) with treating trigger points. I attended the class in 1991, taught by Jeanne Aland at Heartwood Institute, and it completely changed my approach to treating patients. Once I learned about referral patterns, I was able to consistently resolve chronic pain problems.

Over my years of treating thousands of patients, I have added my own observations to those of Doctors Travell and Simons, and developed a variety of self-help techniques, which are included in my books.

In 1999, I received my master's degree in acupuncture. Since then I've been writing trigger point books and articles, teaching trigger point continuing education classes to health care providers, and specializing in treating pain syndromes by combining dry-needling of trigger points with Traditional Chinese Medicine diagnosis and treatment.

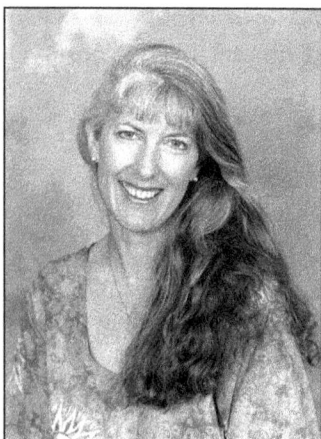

Valerie DeLaune, LAc

Chapter 1: Locating and Treating Trigger Points: General Guidelines

Where to Start?

Chapter 2 contains the *Trigger Point Location Guide;* this will help you figure out which muscles in this book may harbor trigger points that might be causing your symptoms. Locate your pain or other symptoms for each area, and then refer to the chapters listed.

Each muscle chapter has drawings that show the most common pain referral areas for each trigger point. The more solid black or white area indicates the primary area of referral, which is almost always present, and the lighter stippled area shows the most likely secondary areas of referral, which may or may not be present. Keep in mind that the referral patterns only show the most *common* referral patterns; your referral pattern may be somewhat different or even completely different. You may also have overlapping referral patterns from trigger points in multiple muscles. These areas may be more extensive than the patterns common for individual muscles, and pain may be more intense. For this reason, over time, be sure to search for trigger points in all the muscles that refer pain to that area.

Each muscle chapter contains an anatomical drawing of the muscle or muscles covered in that chapter, with "X"'s showing some of the most common locations of trigger points. *There may be additional trigger points or they may be in different places, so search the entire muscle.* Keep in mind that for some muscles, the "X" may just be an *example* of a trigger point location and its associated referral pattern, but they may occur at any level; for example, trigger points in the *paraspinal* muscles.

Each muscle chapter also includes lists of common symptoms and factors that may cause or perpetuate trigger points. Again, these are only the most common; you may experience different symptoms, and your causes and perpetuating factors may be different. If you think you might have trigger points in a certain muscle but don't see any perpetuating factors that apply to you, try to imagine whether anything in your life is similar to something on the list that could be causing the same type of stress on the muscle.

Once you've determined which two muscles most closely fit your pain referral pattern and symptoms, start doing the self-help pressure and stretching, and eliminate the applicable perpetuating factors. Over the next several weeks, search for trigger points in additional muscles, and add those into your treatment regime as needed. As you start to feel better, you'll develop a clearer picture of which trigger points are causing your pain, and which perpetuating factors are reactivating your trigger points.

Other Things to Consider...

When you apply pressure to the trigger point, you can often reproduce the referred pain or other symptoms, but being unable to reproduce the referred pain or other symptoms by applying pressure does *not* rule out involvement of that specific trigger point. Try treating the trigger points that could be causing the problem anyway, and if you improve, even temporarily, assume that one of the trigger points you worked on is indeed at least part of the problem. For this reason, don't work on all the possible trigger points in one session, since you won't know which trigger point treated actually gave you relief.

Be aware that a *primary*, or *key*, trigger point can cause a *satellite* trigger point to develop in a different muscle. The satellite trigger point may have formed for one of these reasons: it lies within the referral zone of the primary trigger point, or it's in a muscle that is either substituting for, or is countering tension for the muscle that contains the primary trigger point. When doing self-treatments, be aware that if some of your trigger points are satellite trigger points, you won't get lasting relief until the primary trigger points have been treated. This is why it is important to work in the direction of referral (see "Do's" below).

You also need to be aware that central sensitization (explained in Appendix B) can cause the referral pattern to deviate from the most common pattern found in each muscle chapter. It may also cause trigger points in several muscles within a region to refer pain to the same area, making it more difficult to determine trigger point locations. This means you can't absolutely rule out the role of a potential trigger point based *only* on consideration of common referral patterns, since other factors may cause you to have an *uncommon* referral pattern. The more intense the earlier pain, the more intense the emotions associated with it, and the longer pain has lasted, the more likely central sensitization will cause deviation from the most common referral patterns.

A small percentage of people will get worse before they get better, mostly in complex cases. Or the pain may move around, or you may have the perception that the pain moved around only because the most painful areas have improved and now you are noticing the next most painful area more. I've only had a few cases where I wasn't able to help patients, because they were so frustrated after receiving little or no help from professional after professional that they only allowed me to treat them a few times before giving up, *even if they had improved*. If you get a little worse before you get better, you may be inclined to give up in the initial stages of treatment. I encourage you to give any treatment you try some amount of time before you decide it isn't working, even if your condition initially gets worse.

General Guidelines for Applying Self-Pressure

DON'Ts:

- **Do not apply pressure over varicose veins, open wounds, infections, herniated/bulging disks, areas of phlebitis/thrombophlebitis, or where clots are present or could be present. If you are pregnant, do not apply pressure on your legs.**

- **Most importantly: *Don't overdo the self-help techniques!*** Many people think that if some feels great, more will be even better, but you can actually make yourself worse by not following the guidelines. Expect gradual improvement, though you may improve most quickly during the initial weeks of therapy.

DO's:

- **Use a tennis ball, racquetball, golf ball, dog play ball, or baseball, or use your elbow or hand if instructed for particular muscles.** For balls, use the weight of your body to give you the pressure; don't press your back or limb onto the balls. The muscle you are working on should be as passive as possible. Use one ball at a time on your back, not one on each side.

- **Apply pressure for a minimum of eight seconds, and a maximum of one minute;** less than eight seconds may activate trigger points, and more than a minute will cut off the circulation for too long and make it worse. Time yourself first to be sure you are actually counting seconds at the correct speed.

- **It should be somewhat uncomfortable, or "hurt good," but it should not be so painful that you are either tensing up or holding your breath. If it is too painful, use a smaller or softer ball, or move to a softer surface (like a bed, or pad your surface with a pillow or blanket).** If it does *not* hurt at all, keep looking for tender spots, or try moving to a harder surface. If it's too tender to lie on, try putting a ball in a long sock and leaning against the wall. I only recommend using the wall if you cannot lie on the ball, since you are then using the very muscles you are trying to work on. You may need to use a combination of surfaces depending on the tenderness of different areas. Over time, as sensitivity decreases, you may need to change ball dimensions and/or hardness, or move to a harder surface.

- **Search the *entire* muscle for tender points, particularly the points of maximum tenderness.** Use the pictures to make sure you are getting the entire muscle and not just the worst spot. Many times a tendon attachment will hurt because the tight muscle is pulling on it, but if you don't treat the bulk of the muscle, it will keep pulling on the attachment.

- **Be sure to work on both sides of the body to keep the muscles balanced, but spend more time on the areas that need it more.** Except for very new one-sided injuries, the same muscle on the opposite side will almost always be tender with pressure, even if it has not yet started causing symptoms. If you loosen one side but not the other, it can lead to additional problems. Sometimes problems with the muscles on the opposite side are actually causing the symptoms, so it is always worth working on both sides.

- **Work in the direction of referral.** For example, if your shoulder hurts and the pain is being referred from trigger points in the trapezius muscle in the upper back, work on the trapezius first, then the infraspinatus and/or supraspinatus, then the deltoid muscles.

- If you have limited time, **do one area thoroughly rather than rushing through many areas**. You are more likely to aggravate trigger points rather than inactivate them if you rush.

- **Do stretches *after* the trigger point work.** If you only have time to do one thing, do the ball/pressure work and skip the stretches.

- **Most people should work on their muscles one time per day initially**. If you have an appointment with your therapist, do not do your self-help the same day. If you are sore from your therapy appointment or your self-help, skip a day. If you are sore for more than one day or your symptoms get worse, it is likely that either the pressure was too hard or you held points for too long. Review these guidelines if that is the case. Tell your therapist if you are sore from their work. This is *not* a case of where if some is great, more is better.

  Pick a time when you will remember to do your self-help, i.e., when you wake up, when you watch television, or when you go to bed, and keep your balls by the bed (*but do not fall asleep on a ball!*).

  After a few weeks, you may wish to increase your self-help to twice per day, as long as you are not getting sore. If a particular activity bothers you, you may wish to do the self-help before and after the activity. If you start getting sore or your symptoms get worse, decrease your self-help frequency.

  Treat your trigger points for as long as they are sensitive, even if active symptoms have disappeared. If trigger points are still tender, they are *latent*, and could easily be reactivated. Most likely you will start forgetting as symptoms disappear; however, the most important thing you will have learned is what to do if your symptoms return.

- **If you have questions or your symptoms get worse, or you are sore for more than one day, stop the self-help until you have had a chance to consult with your therapist**. They should be able to help you figure out any problems.

- **Take your balls on trips with you**, since travel frequently aggravates trigger points. You may even wish to keep some balls at work.

General Guidelines for Stretches and Conditioning

It is very important to distinguish the difference between *stretching* and *conditioning* exercises. *Stretching* means you gently lengthen the muscle fibers. *Conditioning* means you are trying to strengthen the muscle. Doctors Travell and Simons found that *active* trigger points benefited from stretching, but were usually aggravated by conditioning exercises. Once trigger points have been *inactivated*, conditioning is beneficial. Make sure your physical therapist or physiotherapist is familiar with trigger points, and begins your therapy with stretching exercises.

Usually two weeks of trigger point self-help treatment will be sufficient before adding in conditioning exercises, but if your trigger points are still very irritable, you will need to wait until your symptoms improve. Meanwhile, learn the stretches in this book. If you are not sure whether an assigned activity is a stretch or conditioning, ask your practitioner. I will not cover guidelines for conditioning exercises in depth here, since your physical therapist or physiotherapist will prescribe them.

DON'Ts:

- **Don't bounce on stretches, and avoid stretching when your muscles are tired or cold.**

- **Don't do a conditioning exercise just because it worked for someone else.** Doctors Travell and Simons said "Exercise should be regarded as a prescription, much as one prescribes medication. Like a drug, there is a right kind, dose, and timing of exercise." Often a friend will recommend an exercise that worked for them, but you are a different person with a different set of symptoms, and you should no more do their assigned exercises than you would take their prescribed medications. Be sure to tell your therapist all of the activities and exercises/stretches you are doing, because one of these can be contributing to your trigger point activation.

- **Don't keep doing an exercise or stretch that is aggravating your symptoms.** Check with your therapist to determine why it is bothering you and to find out how to proceed.

DO's:

- **Stretch slowly, and only to the point of just getting a gentle stretch; *don't force it*.** If you stretch the muscles too hard or too fast, you can aggravate trigger points.

- **Hold your stretch for 30 to 60 seconds.** There will be little benefit after 30 seconds, but it will not hurt you to stretch for longer either. You may repeat the stretch after releasing and breathing.

- **For any type of repetitive exercise, breathe and rest between each cycle of the exercise.**

- **If you are sore for more than one day** from exercises or stretches, reduce the number of repetitions and try again after the soreness has disappeared. If you are still sore for two days after the exercise or stretch, it needs to be changed.

General Guidelines for Muscle Care

These are some general suggestions for taking care of your muscles; each muscle chapter will have specific suggestions.

DON'Ts:

- Never put the maximum load on a muscle -- it is too easy to strain it.

- Don't lift something too heavy -- ask for help.

- Don't keep muscles in positions of sustained contractions, where you are holding them tense or in sustained use. In order to increase blood flow and bring oxygen and nutrients to the muscles, they need to alternately constrict and relax.

- Don't sit for too long in one position.

- Don't expose your muscles to cold drafts.

DO's:

- After treatments, gently use the muscle in a normal way that uses its full range-of-motion, but avoid strenuous activities immediately afterward or until the trigger points aren't so easily aggravated, whichever is longer.

- Vary your activities so you are not doing any one thing for too long. Rest and take breaks frequently from any given activity.

- Lift with your knees bent and your back straight, with the object close to your chest.

- Notice where you hold tension and practice relaxing those areas.

- Swimming is generally a good exercise, and bicycling is easier on the body than running, but in both cases, take care to avoid straining the trapezius and neck muscles. A recumbent, stationary, or other bike that allows you to sit more upright is preferable.

- When starting an exercise program, *underestimate* what you will be able to do. Gradually add increments in duration, rate, and effort, and in amounts that will not cause you to be sore or activate trigger points.

- Warm-up adequately for sports activities.

- If you are working with a practitioner, they should be able to help you prioritize what needs to be done in order of most importance. If your practitioner is giving you too many things to do at once, be sure to tell them that you are overwhelmed and need to set priorities. Giving a patient too many assignments is all too easy for a practitioner to do, especially when they are first out of school and brimming with many useful ideas and suggestions.

Be sure to return to this chapter often to review the guidelines to ensure you are treating the muscles properly, particularly if something is not working for you, or trigger points are getting aggravated instead of inactivated. Chances are you have forgotten to follow these guidelines.

Be sure to set realistic goals. Focus on a few muscles at a time unless there is a reason that you need to work on several together. Setting unrealistic goals can discourage you, and cause you to give up. It's better to pick just a few things and do them well rather than rush through too many self-help techniques or suggestions and do them poorly. You probably won't be able to apply pressure on five different muscles and stretch them, get orthotics and replace bad shoes, change your diet, and start walking every day all in the first week. Pace yourself so that this is an enjoyable process, and work on the perpetuating factors over time.

Chapter 2: Trigger Point Location Guide

To figure out which muscles to work on first, look at the trigger point location guides and refer to the chapters listed for each. Examine the photos of referral patterns in each chapter and try to find those that most closely match your pain pattern, and read the list of symptoms for each muscle. Refer to chapter 1 for additional instructions on locating and treating trigger points, and general guidelines for applying pressure, stretching, and general muscle care.

1. Scalene (7)
   Levator scapula (6)
   Supraspinatus (11)
   Trapezius (3)
   Multifidi (4)
   Rhomboid (5)
   Triceps (18)
   Biceps (19)

2. Scalene (7)
   Latissimus dorsi (13)
   Levator scapula (6)
   Paraspinals (4)
   Rhomboid (5)
   Serratus posterior superior (10)
   Infraspinatus (12)
   Trapezius (3)

3. Deltoid (17)
   Levator scapula (6)
   Scalene (7)
   Infraspinatus (12)
   Supraspinatus (11)
   Pectoralis Major / Subclavius (8)
   Pectoralis Minor (9)
   Teres major (15)
   Teres minor (16)
   Subscapularis (14)
   Serratus posterior superior (10)
   Latissimus dorsi (13)
   Triceps (18)
   Biceps (19)
   Coracobrachialis (20)

Muscle chapters for all of the remaining areas of the body can be found in *Pain Relief with Trigger Point Self-Help.* Please see the end of this book for more information.

Blank Body Chart

You may wish to make copies of the following blank body chart and draw your symptom pattern on one of them with a colored marker. Then you can compare your pattern with the pain referral pictures in chapters 3 through 20. Out to the side of each painful area, note your pain intensity on a scale of 1 to 10 and the percent of time you feel pain in that area—for example, 6.5/80%. (If you are unable to print from your device, go to http://triggerpointrelief.com/pain_guides.html for a copy you can print off.)

I recommend that you fill out a body chart at least a couple of times per week. Date them so that you'll be able to keep them in order. This chronological record will come in handy in several ways. It will:

- make it easier for you to discern which patterns fit your pain referral most closely;
- help you recognize the factors that cause and perpetuate your symptoms by matching fluctuations in the level and frequency of your symptoms;
- allow you to track your progress (or lack thereof) and provide a historical record of any injuries.

As your condition improves, you may forget how intense your symptoms were originally, and you may think you're not getting any better. You'll be able to see that you are improving, even if you have an occasional setback. One thing to note, however, is that not everyone can accurately draw their pain location, due in part to lack of familiarity with anatomy, so take that possibility into consideration and check muscles with adjacent referral patterns just in case your drawing is inaccurate.

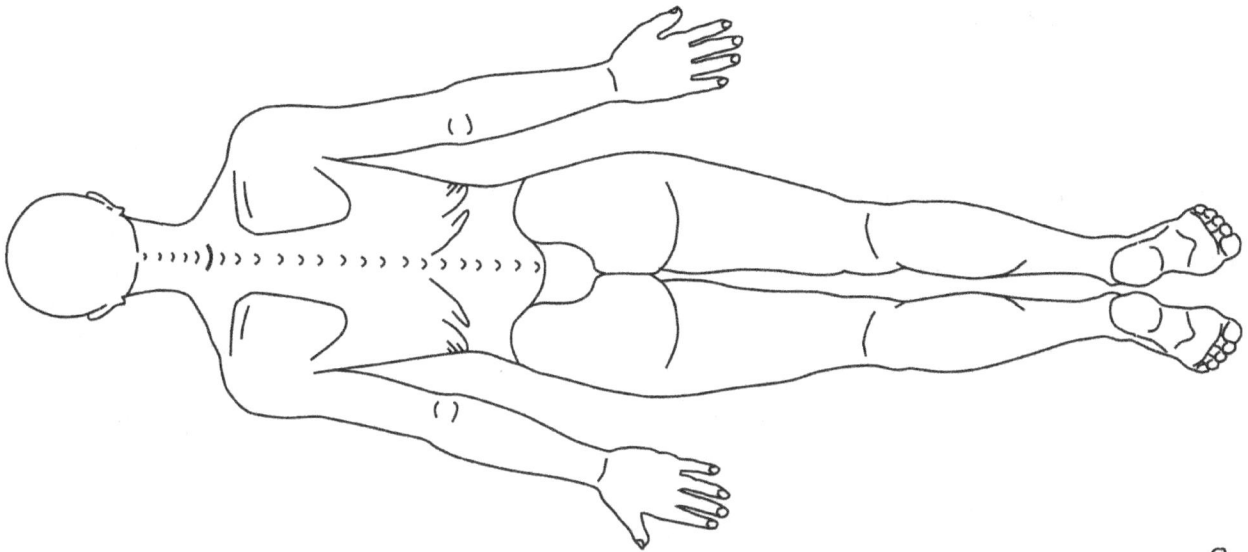

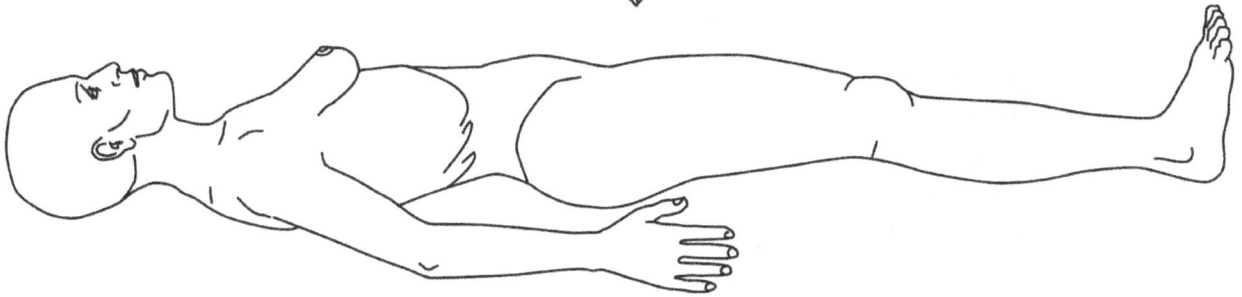

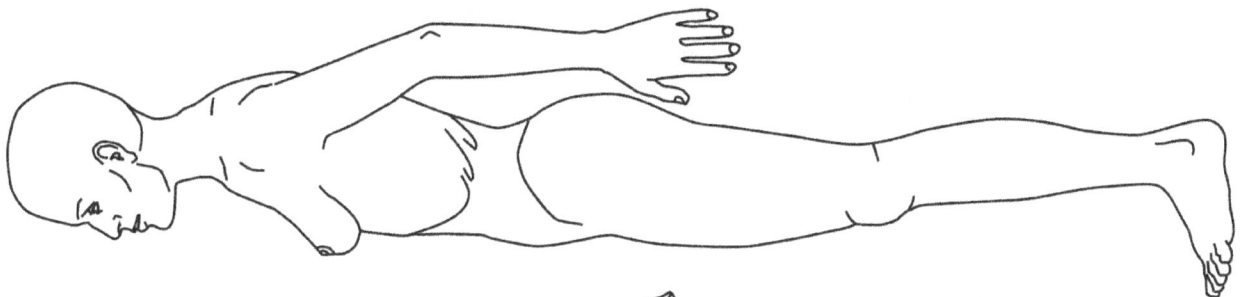

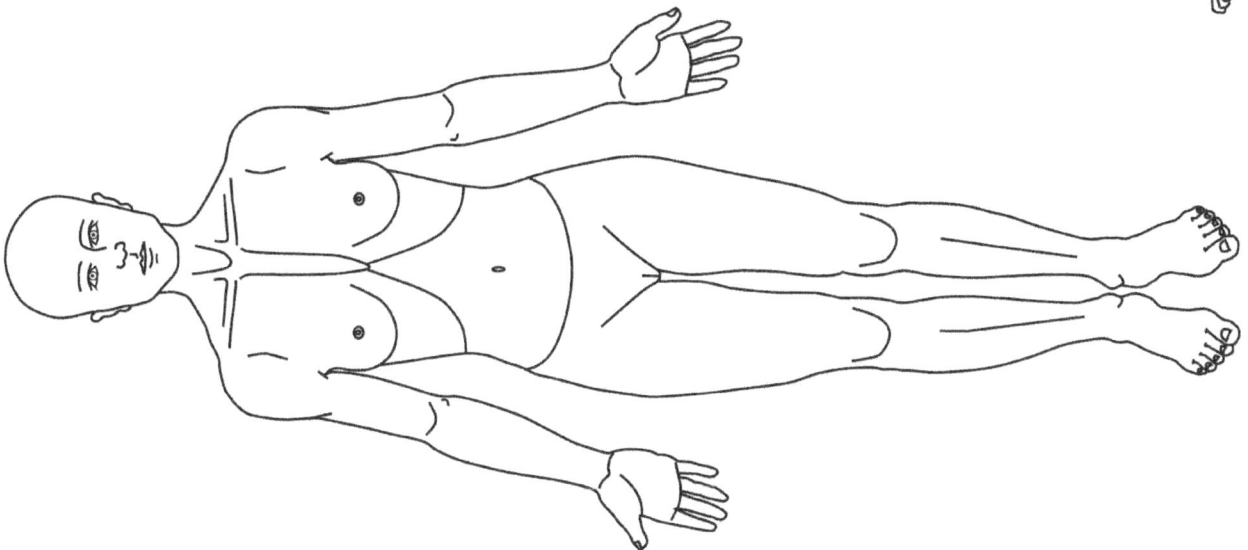

Frozen Shoulder

Trigger points in the *subscapularis* muscle (chapter 14) primarily cause severe painful restriction of motion, and the diagnosis of *frozen shoulder, adhesive capsulitis*, or *hemiplegia* is often used. These are general terms used to describe shoulder pain and restriction of movement, and are usually not a specific diagnosis of what is actually going on physiologically in the shoulder girdle. As symptoms get worse, the patient can't lift their arm above shoulder level and can't reach across their chest. Pain is constant whether using or resting the arm, but is worse with movement and at night. As trigger points in other muscles become involved, they each add their own pain patterns and restriction of movement.

Sometimes thickened tissues are found in the shoulder girdle area in the muscles, the synovial capsule, bursa, or ligaments, but the problem still likely began with trigger points in the *subscapularis* muscle. In fact, trigger points in the *subscapularis* muscle can cause blood vessels to constrict, decreasing the amount of oxygen reaching the muscle cells, and can subsequently actually *form* fibrous, or thickened, tissues in adjacent muscles and lead to *true* adhesive capsulitis. *Subscapularis* trigger points and any trigger points in the surrounding affected muscles must be treated in order for therapy to be effective. The other muscles that typically get involved with the *subscapularis* in a frozen shoulder are the *pectoralis major* (chapter 8), *latissimus dorsi* (chapter 13), *supraspinatus* (chapter 11), and *teres major* (chapter 15).

I strongly encourage you to share the information found in this book with your practitioner; often this condition is treated too aggressively in the initial stages, causing increased pain and involvement of additional muscles. If you do the self-help for all of the muscles in this book, you will likely get a great deal of relief, or complete relief. I definitely recommend trying other techniques before considering surgery, unless an MRI or other imaging test has determined that muscles, tendons, or ligaments are seriously torn or detached, in which case surgery is necessary.

Rotator Cuff Injuries

The *subscapularis* (chapter 14), *supraspinatus* (chapter 11), *infraspinatus* (chapter 12), and *teres minor* (chapter 16) are the four muscles that form the *rotator cuff*. Unfortunately, all too often, pain felt in the shoulder area is diagnosed as a rotator cuff injury without investigating the cause of the pain. A rotator cuff tear must be diagnosed by an MRI, arthrogram, or ultrasound, and it is helpful to know which muscle or muscles contain the tear.

Pain is more often due to trigger points in one of those areas. Even if a tear is confirmed, trigger points may also be present, especially if tightness in the muscle contributed to the overload that led to the tear.

Thoracic Outlet Syndrome

For information on thoracic outlet syndrome, see *scalenes*, chapter 7.

Chapter 3: Trapezius

The *trapezius* commonly contains trigger points, and referred pain from these trigger points is one of the most common pain-related problems. As you can see from the picture, the *trapezius* is a large kite-shaped muscle, covering much of the back and posterior neck.

There are three main parts to the muscle: the upper, middle, and lower *trapezius*, and each part has its own actions and common symptoms.

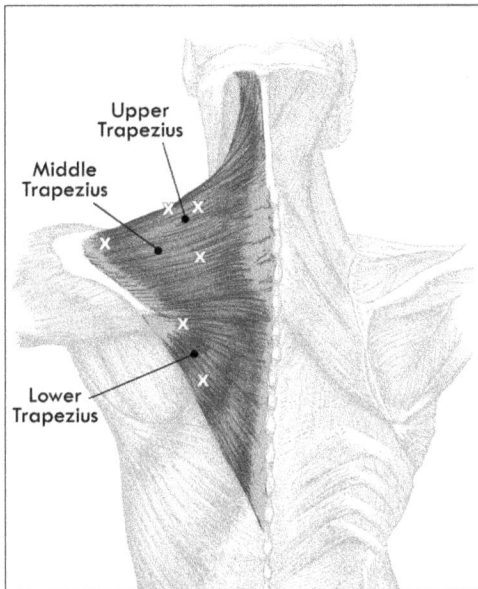

View of upper back

Common Symptoms

Upper Trapezius (TrP 1)
- headaches on the temples / "tension" headaches
- facial, temple, or jaw pain
- pain behind the eye
- dizziness or vertigo (in conjunction with the *sternocleidomastoid* muscle)
- severe neck pain
- a stiff neck
- limited range-of-motion
- intolerance to weight on your shoulders

Middle Trapezius
- mid-back pain
- headaches at the base of your skull
- TrP5 refers superficial burning pain close to the spine
- TrP6 refers aching pain to the top of the shoulder near the joint

Lower trapezius

- mid-back, neck, and/or upper shoulder region pain
- possibly referral on the back of your shoulder blade, down the inside of the arm, and into the ring and little fingers (TrP7), very similar to a *serratus posterior superior* referral pattern (chapter 10)
- headaches at the base of the skull
- TrP3 can refer a deep ache and diffuse tenderness over the top of your shoulder

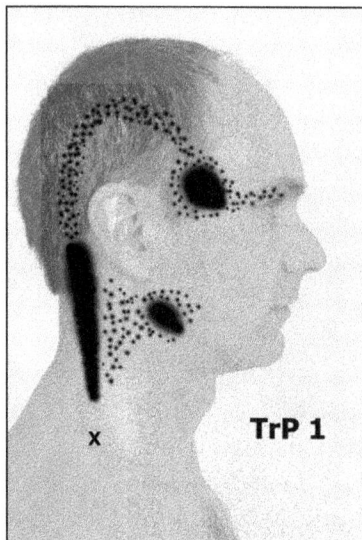

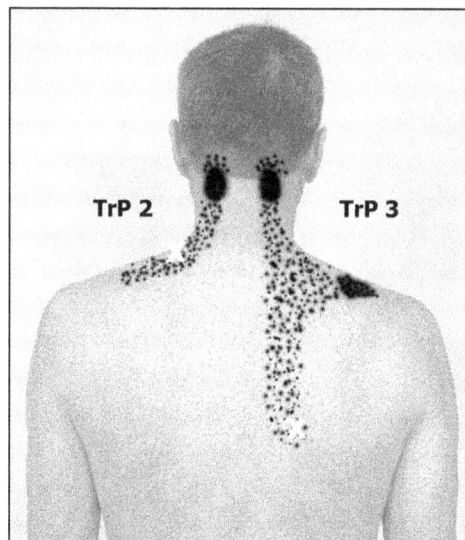

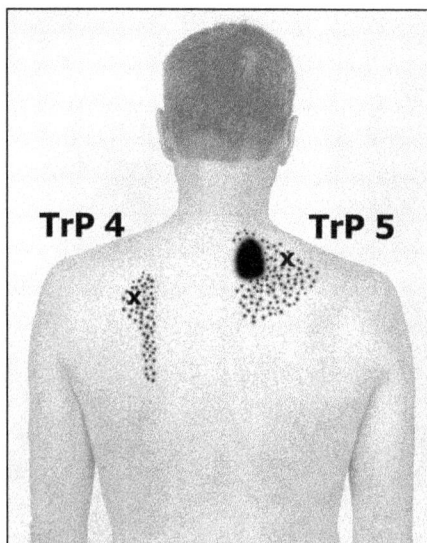

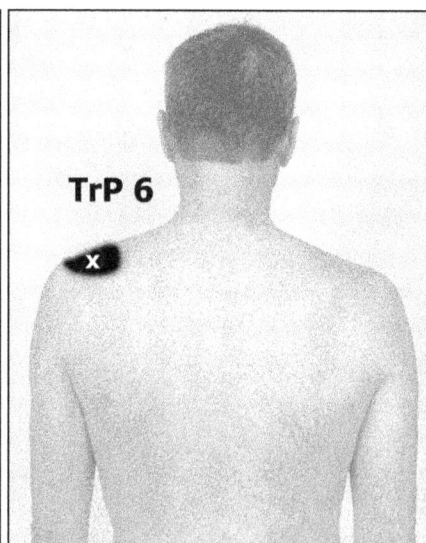

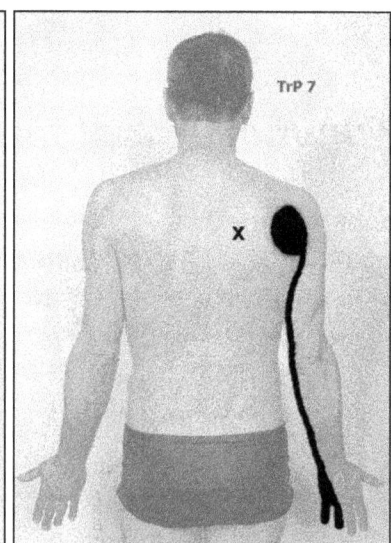

Causes and Perpetuation of Trigger Points

- tensing your shoulders
- cradling a phone between your ear and shoulder
- a chair without armrests, or the armrests are too high
- typing with a keyboard too high
- sitting without a firm back support (sitting slumped)
- turning your head to one side for long periods to have a conversation

- any profession or activity that requires you to bend over for extended periods (i.e.. dentists/hygienists, architects/draftsmen, and secretaries/computer users)
- sewing on your lap with your arms unsupported
- sleeping on your front or back with your head rotated to the side for a long period
- walking with a cane that is too long
- bra straps that are too tight (either the shoulder straps or the torso strap)
- a purse or daypack that is too heavy, or carrying a day pack or purse over one shoulder -- even if you think you are not hiking up one shoulder, you *are*, no matter how light the item
- a mis-fitting, heavy coat
- playing a violin
- jogging
- sports activities with sudden one-sided movements
- backpacking
- bike-riding
- kayaking
- large breasts
- fatigue
- whiplash (a car accident, falling on your head, or any sudden jerk of the head)
- head-forward posture
- tight *pectoralis major* muscles (chapter 8)
- one leg anatomically shorter than the other
- a hemipelvis that is smaller on one side (either the right or left half of the pelvic bone)
- anatomically short upper arms (which causes you to lean to one side to use the armrests)

This is a list of perpetuating factors specific only to trigger points in this muscle. For a full list of perpetuating factors that can cause and perpetuate trigger points anywhere in the body and which also apply to this muscle, please see "Appendix A" (found at the end of this book), since some may need to be addressed for lasting pain relief.

Helpful Hints
- Modify or replace your mis-fitting furniture. Your knees should fit under your desk, and the chair needs to be close enough that you can lean against your backrest. Your elbows should rest on either your work surface or armrests at the same height. Your elbows and forearms should rest evenly on the armrests. Your computer screen should be directly in front of you, and the copy attached to the side of the screen, so that you may look directly forward as much as possible.
- Get a headset or speaker for your phone, or hold the phone with one hand. Shoulder rests are not adequate.
- Any time you must sit for long periods, take frequent breaks. Setting a timer across the room can ensure that you must get up to turn it off.
- When having a conversation, turn and face the person rather than rotating your head in their direction.

- If you must bend over reading materials or plans (such as a draftsman, engineer, or architect), a tilted work surface will alleviate the mechanical stress to a point, but be sure to take frequent breaks.
- Wear bras that fit properly. If you see elastic marks on your skin after you take your bra off, the straps are too tight. Jogging bras work great for medium or small-breasted women. Have the salesperson help you find a bra that fits properly -- many of them really know their products.
- If you have a foam rubber pillow, get rid of it! Vibrations from these pillows will aggravate trigger points. Your pillow should support your head at a level that is comfortable when you are lying on your side (not too high or too short). I always take my pillow with me when I travel -- I know I have something comfortable to sleep on, and it comes in handy if I get stuck in an airport.
- Wear your daypack over both shoulders. If you carry a purse, get one with a long strap and put the strap over your head, so you are wearing it diagonally across your torso, and keep its contents light. If you backpack, try to put most of the weight on your hip strap.
- Restoration of proper posture, especially head positioning, is critical to treating trigger points since head-forward posture can both cause and perpetuate trigger points. Head-forward posture can be aggravated while sitting in a car, at a desk, in front of a computer, or while eating dinner or watching TV. Using a good lumbar support everywhere you sit will help correct poor sitting posture. See the exercise below in the "Self-Help Techniques" section for postural re-training.

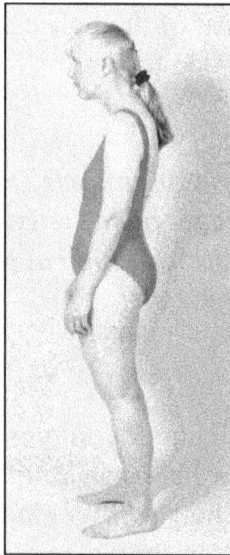 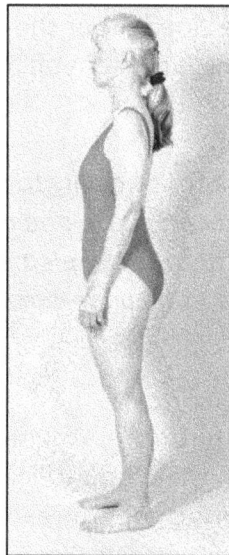

Poor posture   ***Good Posture***

- Putting your hands in your pockets when standing takes the weight off the *trapezius* muscle.
- Putting shoulder pads in a heavy coat can help take the weight off the upper *trapezius*.
- If you have a body asymmetry or short upper arms, see a specialist to get compensating lifts or pads.

- If your breasts are large enough that they cause backaches, your insurance company may cover breast reduction surgery if your doctor recommends it. Carefully consider the risks of surgery if you are considering this option.

Self-Help Techniques

Applying Pressure

Paraspinal / Trapezius Pressure: See chapter 4 for how to use a ball to apply pressure to most of the *paraspinal* muscles and the mid to lower *trapezius* muscle.

Backnobber®: If you are at work and unable to lie on the floor, I recommend using a Backnobber® from Pressure Positive Company to apply pressure to the *trapezius* muscle. Note how both hands are pulling the Backnobber® away from the body in the direction the arrows are pointing, rather than pressing it into the front of the trunk to lever pressure onto the back.

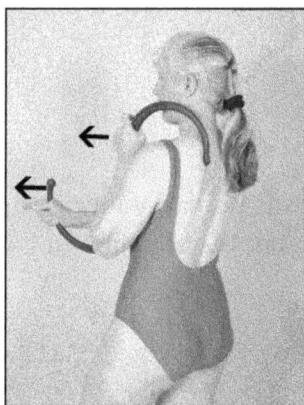

Trapezius Pinch: Place your elbow and forearm on a surface high enough to support the weight of your arm. With the opposite hand, reach across your front and pinch the upper portion of the *trapezius* muscle. Be sure to stay on the meat of the muscle and *do not dig your thumb into the depression directly above the collarbone.* You may need to tilt your head slightly toward the side you are working on, to keep the muscle relaxed enough to be able to pinch it.

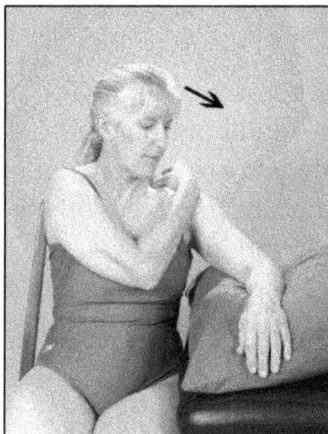

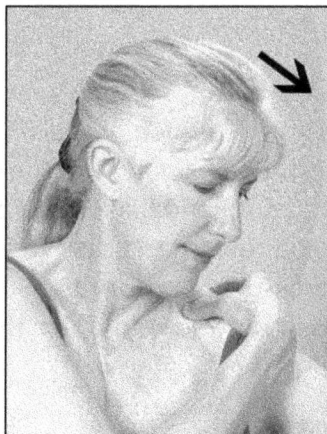

Supraspinatus Pressure: The *supraspinatus* pressure (chapter 11) will also help treat the upper trapezius.

Posterior Neck Pressure: I find it is best to treat the *trapezius* muscles first and the *posterior neck* muscles second.

The shading in the picture marks the area to work on. You may work along the base of the skull and down the back of the neck. Try to get all the way to the base of the neck where it intersects the top of the shoulder, in order to work on the entire *splenius cervicis* muscle.

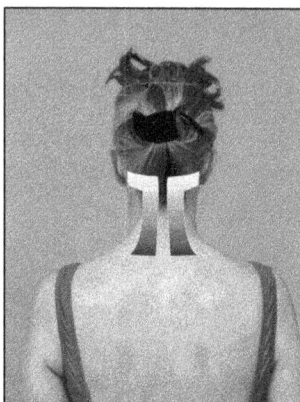

To treat the back of your neck, use a golf ball and lie face-up with your hands behind your neck. One palm should be squarely over the other palm, with the golf ball in the center of your top palm, and *not* where the fingers join the palm.

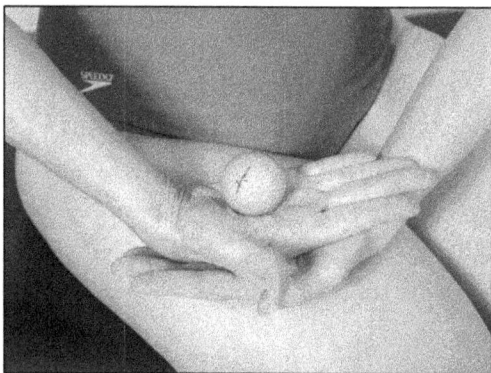

Keep your head relaxed throughout the self-treatment. To apply pressure, rotate your head toward the ball. Be sure to work on the muscles to the *side* of the spine—don't put the ball directly *on* the spine. To move the ball, roll your head away from the side you are working on, move the ball a small amount, and then rotate your head back toward the side you are working on. If you want more pressure, rotate your head toward the side you are working on even more; rotate your head less if you want less pressure. *Do not raise your head to move the ball.* This will cause additional stress on the muscles, so be sure to move the ball by *rotating* your head away from it.

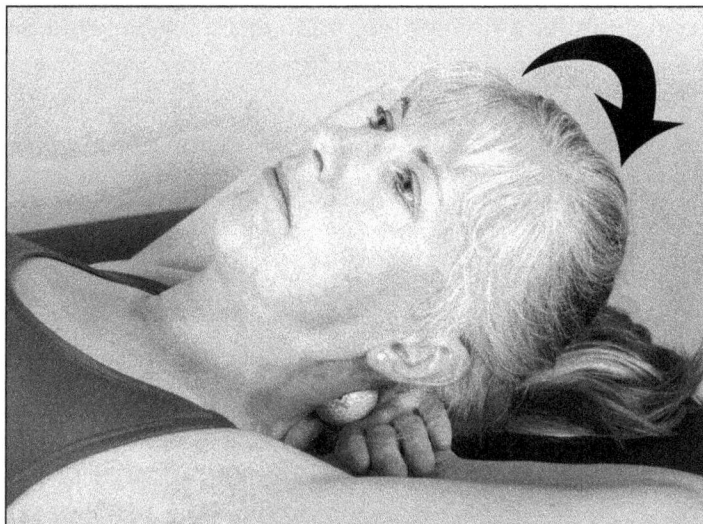

Stretches

Trapezius Stretch: This stretch benefits the middle and lower *trapezius*. Start with your arms at your sides and then move them through the positions indicated in the photographs. End with your arms at your sides and take two deep breaths. Repeat three to five times.

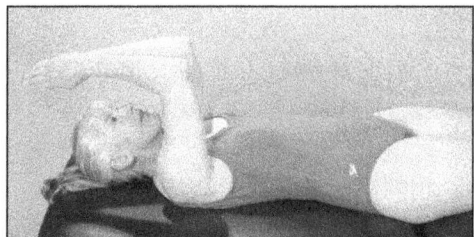

Step 1

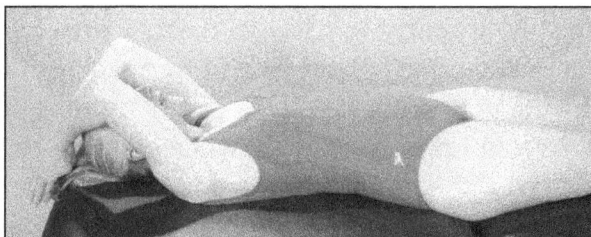

Step 2

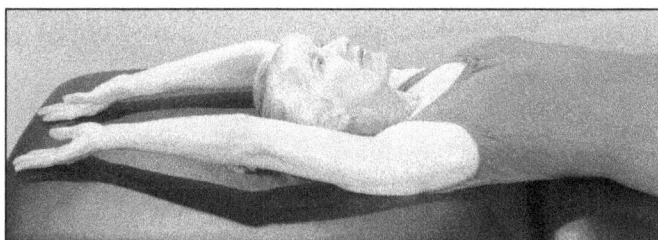

Step 3

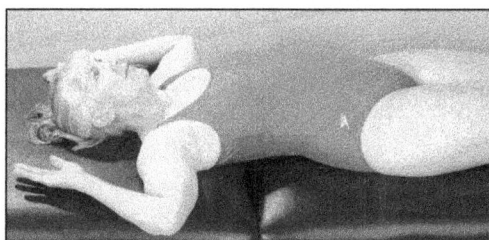

Step 4

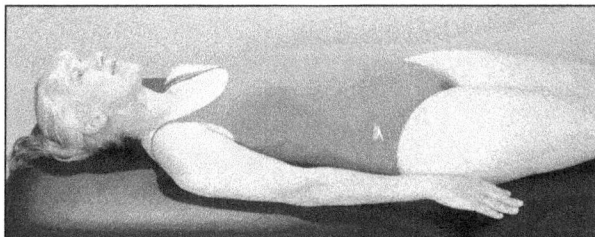

Step 5

Posterior Neck Stretch: You may do this stretch under a hot shower and, if possible, seated on a stool. Lock your fingers behind your head and pull your head gently forward. Turn your head to one side at a 45° angle and gently pull your head in that direction. Place one hand on the top of your head and gently pull your head down to that side. Repeat on the opposite side.

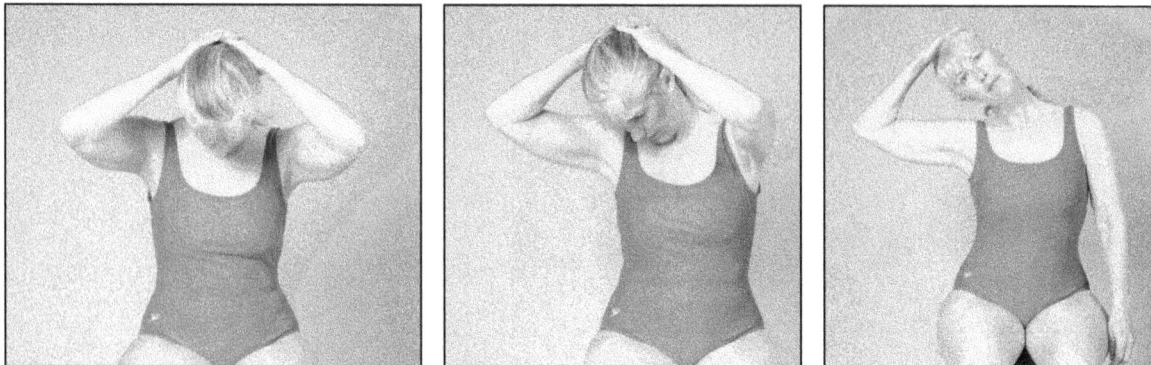

Pectoralis Stretch: The *pectoralis* stretch will benefit the *trapezius* muscle; see chapter 8.

Exercises

Postural Re-training: Postural exercises can help eliminate head-forward posture. To learn proper posture and correct a head-forward position, stand with your feet about four inches apart, with your arms at your sides and thumbs pointing forward. Tighten your buttocks to stabilize your lower back, then, while inhaling, rotate your arms and shoulders out and back by rotating your thumbs backward, and squeeze the shoulder blades together in the back. Keep holding this position while dropping your shoulders down and exhaling. Move your head back to bring your ears in line with your shoulders and hold this position for about six seconds while breathing normally.

When moving your head, don't move your nose up or down, or open your mouth. Relax, but then try to maintain good posture once you release the pose. If holding this position feels uncomfortable or "stiff," try shifting your body weight from your heels to the balls of your feet, which causes your head to move backward over your shoulders. This exercise should be repeated frequently during the day in order to retrain yourself in good postural techniques, at least every one to two hours. It is better to do one repetition six or more times per day than to do six repetitions in a row.

Also See:
*   Supraspinatus (chapter 11)
*   Levator scapula (chapter 6)
*   Rhomboid (chapter 5)
*   Pectoralis major (chapter 8)
*   Pectoralis minor (chapter 9)
*   Infraspinatus (chapter 12)

You may also need to search for trigger points in the *sternocleidomastoid, temporalis* (satellite trigger points), *occipitalis* (satellite trigger points), and/or *masseter* (satellite trigger points), since trigger points in those muscles can either cause similar pain referral patterns or may affect or be affected by *trapezius* trigger points in some way.

Since trigger points in these muscles don't directly cause shoulder pain, they are not addressed in this book. If you can't relieve your pain with the self-help techniques in this book after six to eight weeks, you may wish to consider whether you need to treat trigger points in these additional muscles, or if you still have perpetuating factors to resolve. Go to the end of this book for other books by the author that provide self-treatment techniques of muscles not covered in this book.

Differential Diagnosis: If you are unable to relieve your symptoms with trigger point self-help techniques, you may need to see a health care provider to rule out occipital neuralgia and cervicogenic headaches. Or, you may need to see a chiropractor or osteopathic physician to be evaluated for vertebrae that are out of alignment.

Chapter 4: Paraspinals

(Iliocostalis Lumborum, Iliocostalis Thoracis,
Longissimus Thoracis, Multifidi)

Part of this muscle group runs the entire length of the spine, and some of the muscles run most of the length of the spine. Yet others (the *multifidi*) are small muscles that attach one vertebra to the next. These are the muscles that allow you to bend and twist.

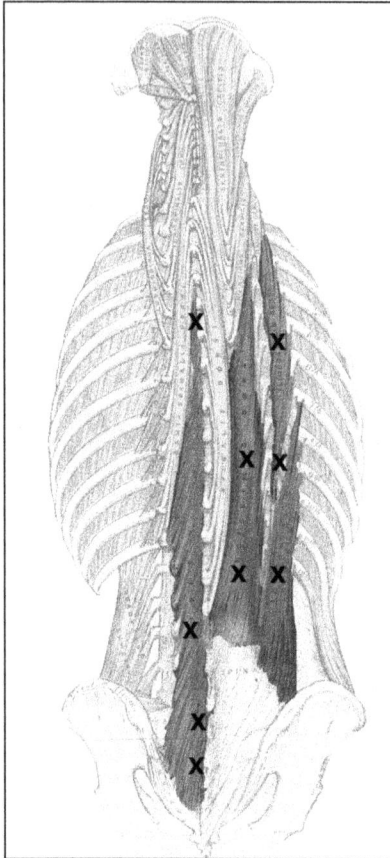

Back view of trunk

Common Symptoms

- See the pictures for all the pain referral patterns. These pictures show common trigger points, **but trigger points can develop <u>at any level</u> and cause similar referral patterns <u>at any level</u>**. Please note that in many cases pain can refer to the front side of the body, causing you to think you are having organ problems, particularly in the area of the heart. Trigger points in these muscles are an often overlooked cause of buttocks pain.
- deep, aching pain that feels like it is in the spine
- pain may increase with coughing or straining to have a bowel movement
- restricted range-of-motion or restricted rotation of the trunk, possibly severe
- possibly difficulty climbing stairs or getting out of a chair
- possibly nausea, belching, and gastrointestinal pain and cramping

- entrapment of spinal nerves cause increased or decreased sensitivity and/or uncomfortable sensations on the skin of the back
- stiffness in the spine, mostly from the *longissimus thoracis*

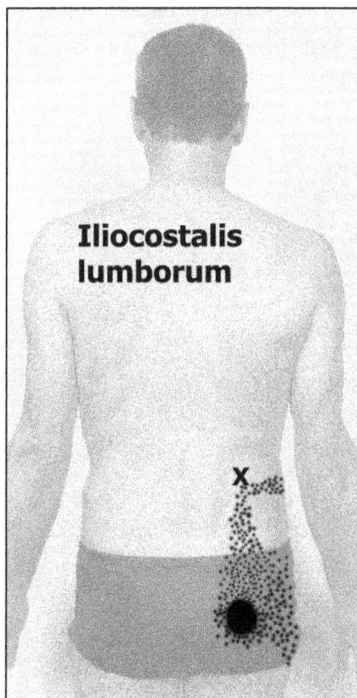

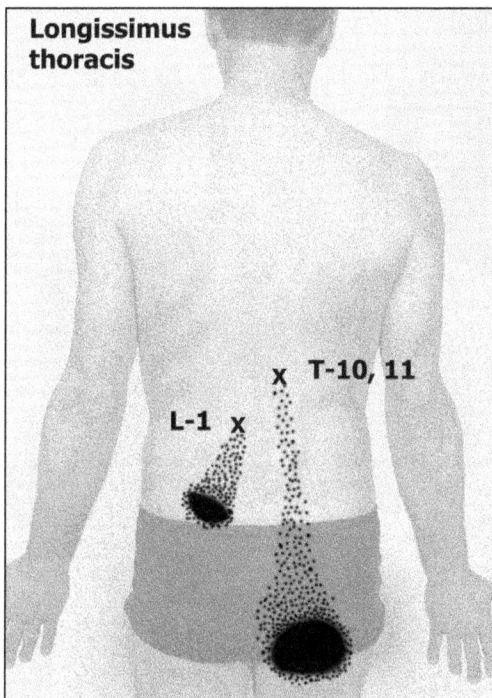

Iliocostalis lumborum

Longissimus thoracis

T-10, 11

L-1

> **Sample referral patterns, but all of these can occur at any level of the back.**

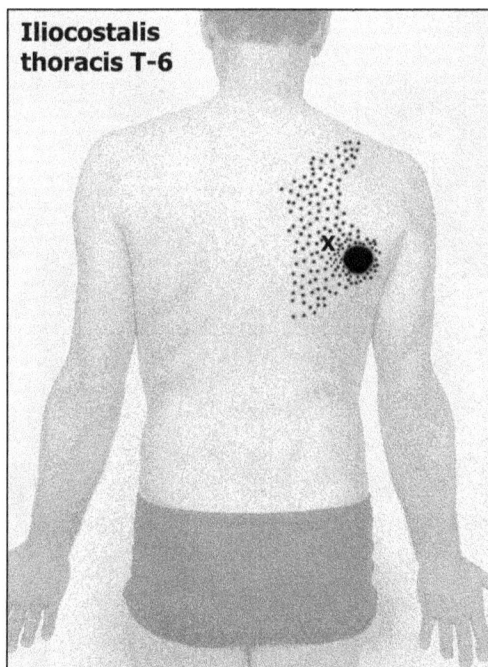

Iliocostalis thoracis T-6

Iliocostalis thoracis T-6

Back referral pattern

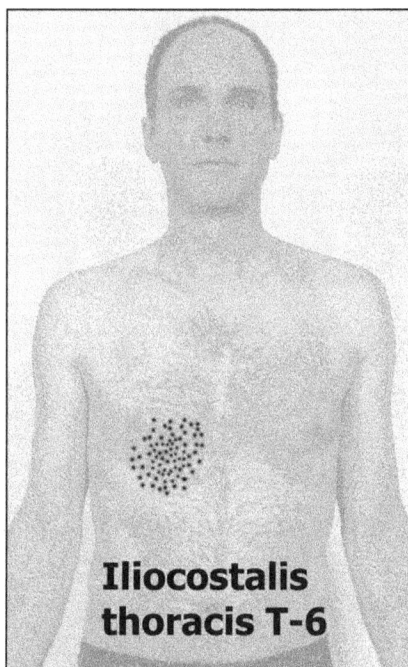

Front referral pattern

Iliocostalis thoracis T-11

Iliocostalis thoracis T-11

Sample referral patterns, but all of these can occur at any level of the back.

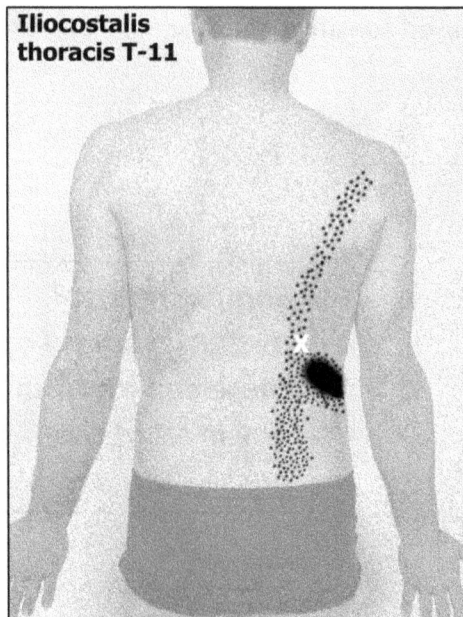

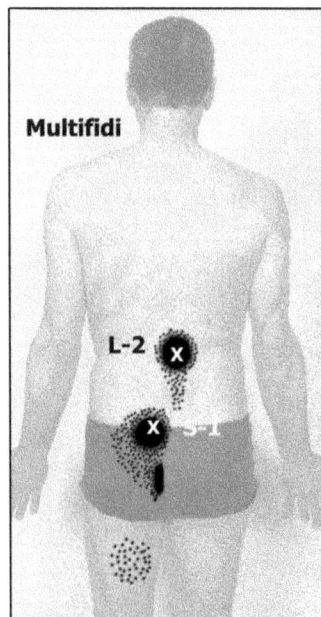

Back referral pattern

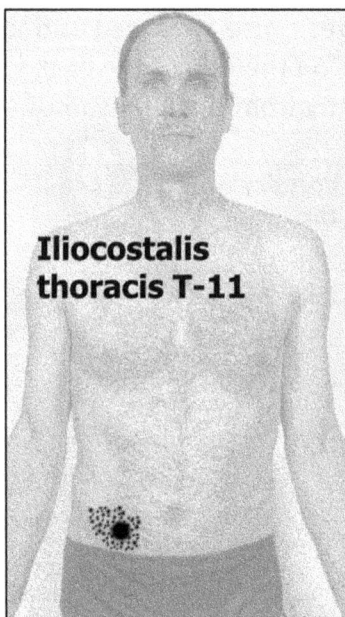

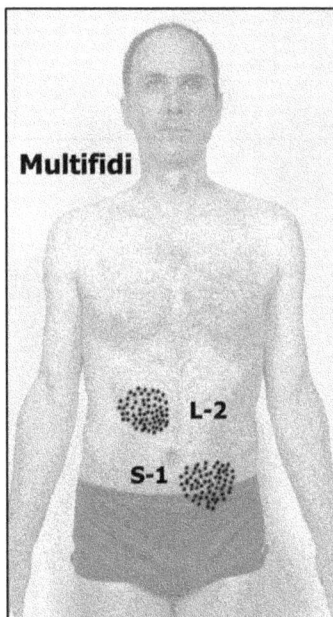

Front referral pattern

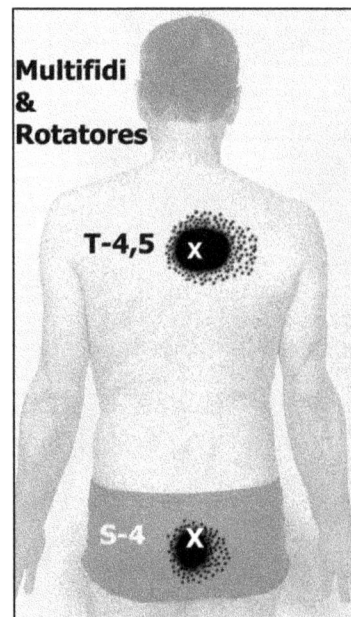

Multifidi

Multifidi

Multifidi & Rotatores

L-2

X

S-1

L-2

S-1

T-4,5 X

S-4 X

Back referral pattern

Front referral pattern

Causes and Perpetuation of Trigger Points

- a sudden overload, often when bending, lifting, and twisting at the same time (people frequently tell me they were moving boxes)
- catching yourself from falling, such as when slipping on ice
- sitting for long periods without moving, in as little as hour or less for some people
- sitting on a wallet in your back pocket
- bending over while gardening
- injury is more likely when the muscles are chilled or fatigued

- car accidents, especially a whiplash injury
- mattresses that are too old or too soft, or sleeping next to someone who is heavier and trying to avoid rolling into them
- a tight belt or bra strap
- trigger points in the *latissimus dorsi* (chapter 13)
- head-forward posture
- one leg anatomically shorter than the other, or an unequal hemipelvis size (either the right or left half of the pelvis)

This is a list of perpetuating factors specific only to trigger points in <u>these</u> muscles. For a full list of perpetuating factors that can cause and perpetuate trigger points anywhere in the body and which also apply to these muscles, please see "Appendix A" (found at the end of this book), since some may need to be addressed for lasting pain relief.

Helpful Hints

- Don't keep a wallet in a back pocket, since it will tilt your pelvis and spine when sitting.
- Modify or replace your mis-fitting furniture. Your knees should fit under your desk, and the chair needs to be close enough that you can lean against your backrest. Your elbows should rest on either your work surface or armrests at the same height. Your elbows and forearms should rest evenly on the armrests. Your computer screen should be directly in front of you, and the copy attached to the side of the screen, so that you may look directly forward as much as possible. Take frequent breaks.
- Get a headset or speaker for your phone, or hold the phone with one hand. Shoulder rests are not adequate.
- If you must bend over plans or reading materials (such as a draftsman, engineer, or architect), a tilted work surface will alleviate the mechanical stress to a point, but be sure to take frequent breaks.
- Lift properly by bending your knees rather than your back, and hold objects close to your body.
- Wear bras that fit properly. If you see elastic marks on your skin after you take your bra off, the straps are too tight. Jogging bras work great for medium or small-breasted women. Have the salesperson help you find a bra that fits properly -- many of them really know their products.
- If you are gardening, straighten up frequently, and stand and stretch periodically.
- Be sure to slide into the center of your car seat. Some bucket seats curve up on each side, and if you are not in the center, your pelvis is tilted.
- Buy a firm mattress, and replace it every five to seven years. You can put plywood between the box springs and mattress to make it firmer.
- If you have difficulty getting up, roll over onto your hands and knees and crawl to where you can grab onto something and pull yourself up.
- When standing up from a chair, slide your butt to the front of the chair, turn your entire body a little sideways, put one foot under the front edge of the chair, then stand with your torso erect so that your thighs take the load. You can use your hands to assist you if necessary. Sit down in the opposite sequence.

- When climbing stairs or a ladder, rotate your entire body 45-degrees and keep your back straight.
- Restoration of proper posture, especially head positioning, is critical to treating trigger points since head-forward posture can both cause and perpetuate trigger points. Head-forward posture can be aggravated while sitting in a car, at a desk, in front of a computer, or while eating dinner or watching TV. Using a good lumbar support everywhere you sit will help correct poor sitting posture.   See *trapezius* (chapter 3) for this exercise.
- If you have a body asymmetry or an anatomically shorter leg, see a specialist to get compensating lifts or pads.

Self-Help Techniques

Applying Pressure

Paraspinal / Trapezius Pressure: The shading on the picture marks the area you will want to work on.

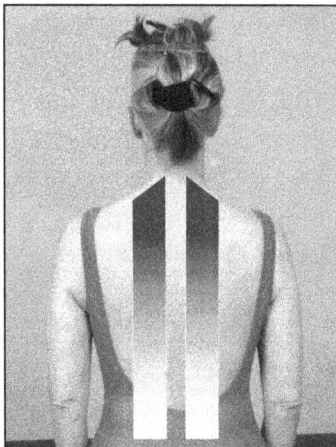

Lie face-up on a firm bed or the floor, with your knees bent. Using a tennis ball or racquet ball, start at the shoulder, about one inch out to the side of the spine, and hold pressure for eight seconds to one minute per spot. Shift a small amount to the next spot further down the back by using your legs to move your body over the ball, and continue to hold pressure on each spot. Continue working down all the way to the top of the pelvis in order to treat both the *trapezius* and the *paraspinal* muscles. You may want to repeat this on a second line further out from the spine, especially if you have a wide back or if you have tender points further out. *Do not do this directly on the spine!* I recommend using one ball at a time, rather than using a ball on each side at the same time. By performing this technique lying down, as opposed to standing and leaning into the wall, you keep the muscles as passive as possible, so that you are not using them to hold you upright while you are applying pressure.

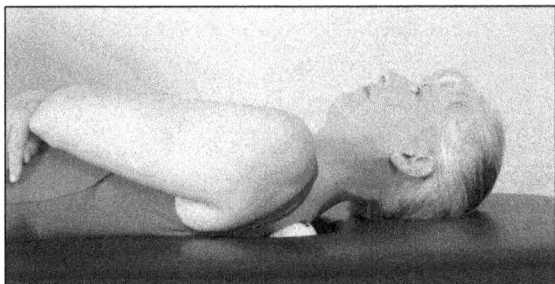

If you are at work and unable to lie on the floor, I recommend using a Backnobber® from Pressure Positive Company (see chapter 3).

Longissimus thoracis pressure: To work on the *longissimus thoracis*, which is very close to the spine, you will need to lie on a hard floor and use a golf ball. Place the golf ball *in between* your spine and the muscle (not *on* the spine—see photo), and then move your body just a little *away* from the side you are working on. This presses on the muscles at a 45° angle, the only really effective way to get this muscle. Do this from the bottom of the neck, down to the top of the pelvis. As a trigger point therapist, I perform this treatment by standing on the opposite side and leaning across, pressing the muscle out at a 45° angle.

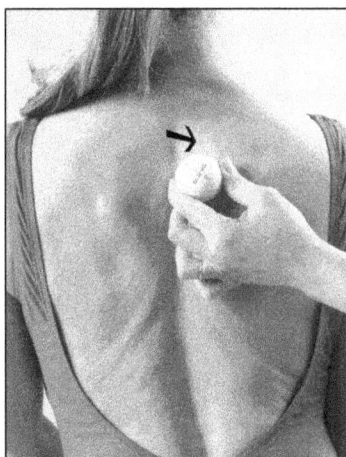

Demonstrating location of muscle and direction to press out against golf ball

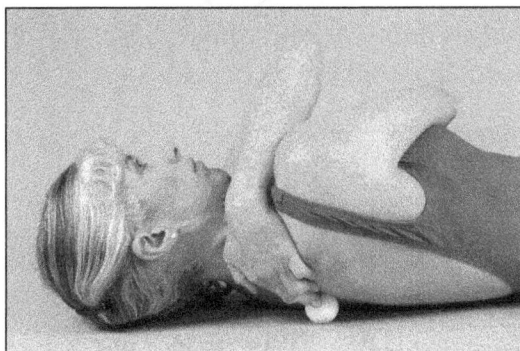

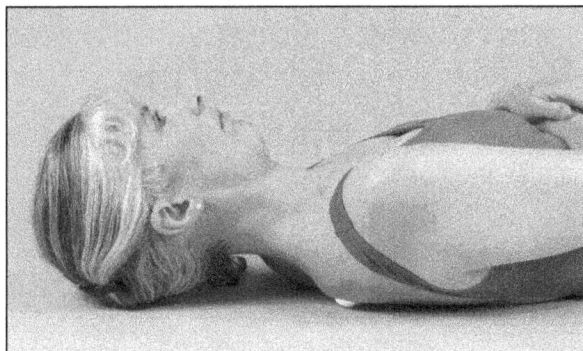

Lay on a golf ball to perform this self-help technique

Multifidi pressure: To treat the *multifidi* (the little muscles that attach one vertebra to the next), you will need the assistance of another person, as even a golf ball is too large. They will need a tool, such as a rubber-tipped wooden dowel (available at a massage supply store), or an eraser that is rounded off. Working next to the spinous process (the pointy part of the vertebra), massage in the groove next to it. Your assistant may be able to use their thumb, but a gadget works better and is easier on the person administering the treatment.

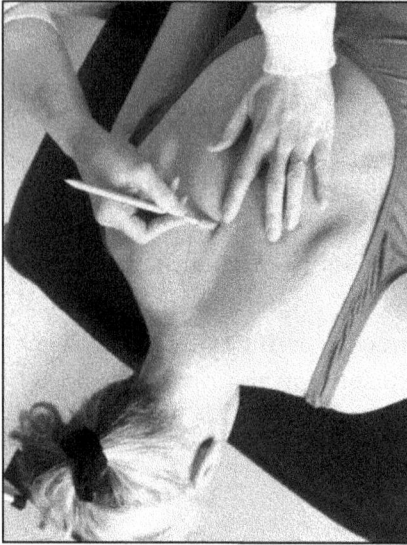

Posterior Neck Pressure: See chapter 5

Stretches

In-Bathtub Stretch: With your head hanging forward, lean forward and reach your hands down toward your toes, until you are feeling a gentle stretch. Relax and then repeat, moving your hands further down each time, but only as far down as you can feel a gentle stretch. Do this in a hot bath if you can. [**Note**: If you have trigger points in the *iliopsoas* muscle, even if they are latent, this stretch can cause a reactive cramp. You may need to work on and stretch the *iliopsoas* first, but since trigger points in the *iliopsoas* muscles don't directly cause shoulder pain, they are not addressed in this book. Go to the end of this book for other books by the author that provide self-treatment techniques of muscles not covered in this book.]

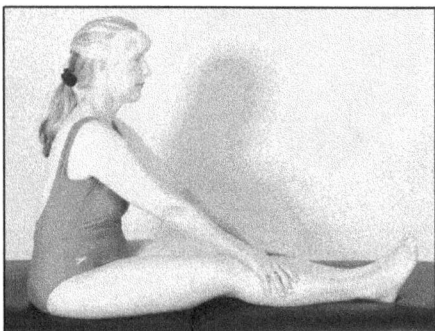

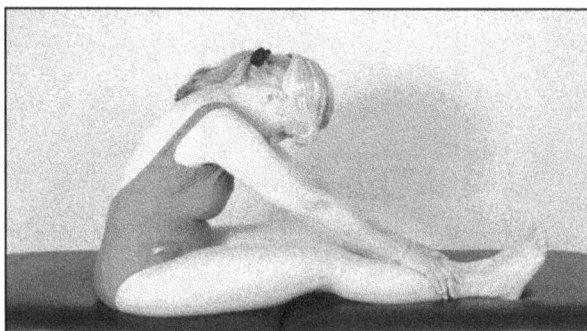

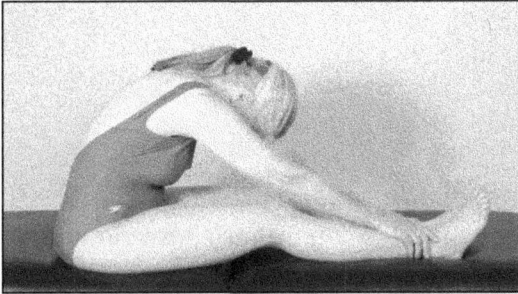

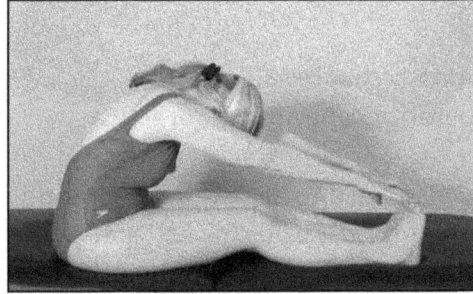

Low Back Stretching Exercise: Lying on your back, with your hands clasped *behind* one knee, gently bring that knee toward your chest until you are just feeling the stretch. Repeat with the opposite knee, and then both legs at the same time.

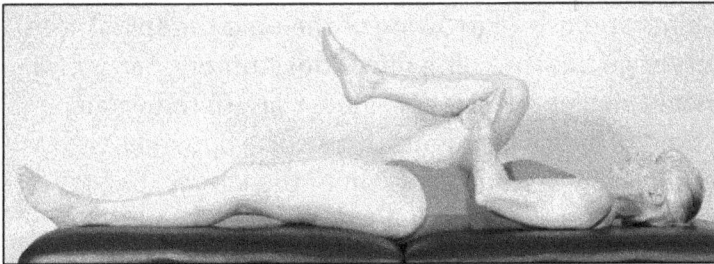

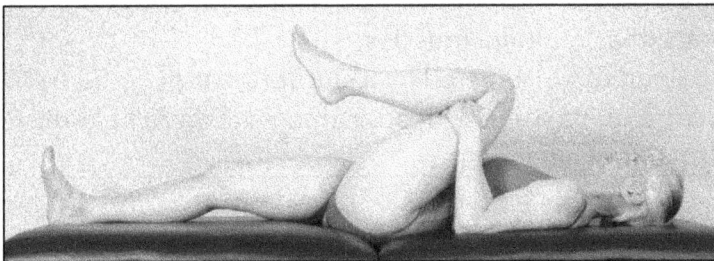

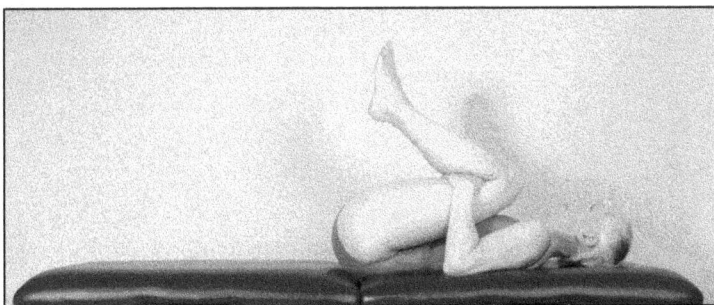

Also See:
* Latissimus dorsi (chapter 13)
* Serratus posterior superior (chapter 10)

You may also need to search for trigger points in the *quadratus lumborum*, *serratus posterior inferior*, and *iliopsoas*, since trigger points in those muscles can either cause similar pain referral patterns or may affect or be affected by *paraspinal* trigger points in some way.

Since trigger points in these muscles don't directly cause shoulder pain, they are not addressed in this book. If you can't relieve your pain with the self-help techniques in this book after six to eight weeks, you may wish to consider whether you need to treat trigger points in these additional muscles, or if you still have perpetuating factors to resolve. Go to the end of this book for other books by the author that provide self-treatment techniques of muscles not covered in this book.

Differential Diagnosis: If you are experiencing pain in the spine, you will need to see a health care provider to rule out herniated discs, spinal stenosis (narrowing of the hole the spinal cord goes through, or of one of the holes the nerves go out through), infections, tumors, cancer, or other more serious problems. Other diagnoses that should be considered are fibromyalgia, organ disease, osteoarthritis, fat lobules, strain of spinal ligaments, retrocecal appendicitis, a dissecting aortic aneurysm or saddle thrombus, kidney stones, torsion of the kidney, pelvic inflammatory disease, endometriosis, ankylosing spondylitis, Paget's disease, leukemia, Hodgkin's disease, prostatitis and seminal vesiculitis, or sacroiliitis. A finding of osteoarthritis in itself may not account for the pain felt, since you can have pain without degenerative changes to the spine, and you can have degenerative changes without pain. Lumbar zygapophysial (facet) joints may refer pain in the same pattern as multifidi muscles.

Vertebrae may be out of alignment and need to be adjusted by a chiropractor or osteopathic physician. Combining acupuncture or massage with adjustments is more helpful, since tight muscles will keep pulling vertebra out of alignment.

Chapter 5: Rhomboid

This muscle attaches on the spine and on the middle edge of the shoulder blade (scapula). Most of the time trigger points are formed in the *rhomboid* muscles due to tight *pectoralis major* and /or *pectoralis minor* muscles. Even though you may not be experiencing the referral patterns of the "pecs," there may be tightness and/or latent trigger points in those muscles that are causing stress on the *rhomboid* muscles.

I find that often health care practitioners want to focus on strengthening the *rhomboids*, rather than eliminating trigger points and tightness in the pectoralis muscles. When working on yourself, it is important to check and work on the pectoralis muscles first, then the *rhomboids* second.

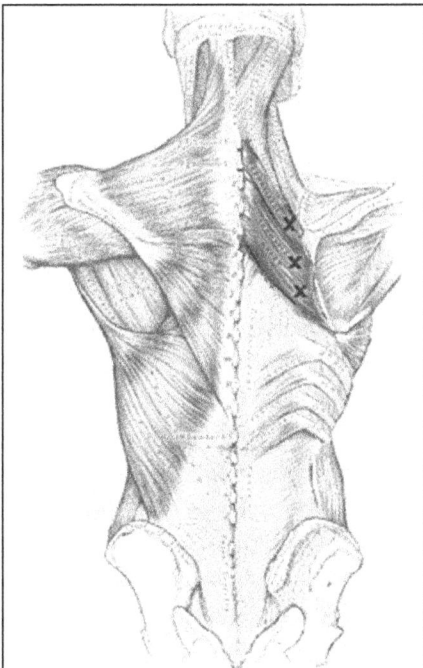
View of back of trunk

Common Symptoms

- pain is usually pretty localized in the mid-back, close to the shoulder blade, and usually feels fairly superficial and achy
- pain may also spread over the top edge of the shoulder blade
- often the shoulder will appear rounded forward, indicative of *pectoralis major* and/or *pectoralis minor* involvement (chapters 8 and 9)
- symptoms may be aggravated by lying on the side of pain, or by reaching forward or stretching to reach something
- snapping and crunching noises during movement of the shoulder blade may be due to trigger points in the *rhomboid* muscle

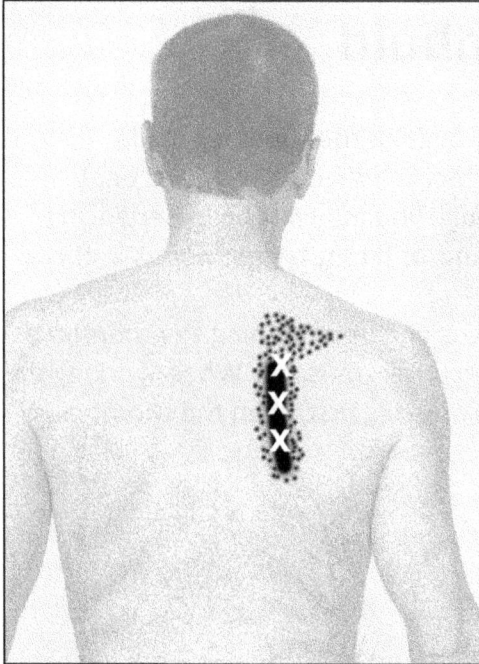

Causes and Perpetuation of Trigger Points

- leaning forward with the shoulders rounded forward for long periods of time, such as when sewing
- holding your arms out for a long time period, such as when painting a ceiling
- tightness or trigger points in the *pectoralis major* and/or *pectoralis minor* muscles (chapters 8 and 9)
- chronic discouragement and/or sadness may cause you to slump your shoulders forward and breathe improperly
- upper thoracic scoliosis (curvature of the spine in the mid to upper back area)

This is a list of perpetuating factors specific only to trigger points in <u>this</u> muscle. For a full list of perpetuating factors that can cause and perpetuate trigger points anywhere in the body and which also apply to this muscle, please see "Appendix A" (found at the end of this book), since some may need to be addressed for lasting pain relief.

Helpful Hints

- Be sure to take frequent breaks if you must sit for long periods. Setting a timer across the room ensures you will get up periodically and relieve pressure on the *rhomboids*.
- A lumbar support helps correct round-shouldered posture. It seems, oddly enough, that most car seats actually *curve the wrong way* in the lumbar area. Most chiropractic offices carry lumbar supports of varying thickness. I recommend getting one for the car and your favorite seat at home, and investing in a good chair for the office, even if your employer won't. Try to avoid sitting in or on anything without back support, which causes you to sit with your shoulders and upper back slumped forward. When going to sporting events, picnics, or other places you won't have a back support, bring a *Crazy Creek Chair* (or something similar) to provide at least some support. You can get one

through most of the major sporting goods suppliers, and they cost about $50, a good investment in your back, and they are very lightweight for carrying. Or consider a lightweight collapsible chair, also available at sporting goods stores.

- Some scoliosis will be corrected with the ball work. Chiropractic care focuses on correcting scoliosis. Corrective orthotics (custom footbeds) may also be necessary to correct muscular imbalances on a permanent basis. If you have an anatomically shorter leg or a small hemipelvis (either the right or left half of the pelvic bone), be sure to see a specialist to get compensating lifts and pads.
- Learn to breathe properly (see *scalenes*, chapter 7).

Self-Help Techniques

Applying Pressure

Pectoralis Pressure: You should apply pressure to the *pectoralis* muscles first before working on the *rhomboid*s; see chapter 8.

Rhomboid Pressure: Use a tennis ball or racquet ball. Lie face-up, and hold your arm across your chest to pull the scapula out of the way and access the trigger points along the edge of the scapula. Then, while leaning over onto the ball with however much pressure you want to apply, work from the top edge of the scapula to the bottom. It is just easier to work in this direction, but not critical. It is also easier to move from spot to spot if your legs are bent, and you shift yourself to the next spot by using your legs to slide your body over the ball, rather than moving the ball with your hand. As you lean onto the ball, be sure not to let your arm drop back down, as this closes up the space next to your shoulder blade, and you will miss some of the worst spots. Patients will often sense they "just can't seem to get to the main spot," so if you think you might be missing the *rhomboid* muscle, check your arm positioning and make sure the ball is close to the edge of the scapula.

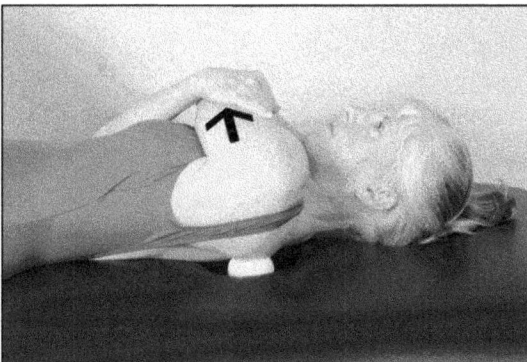

Be sure to also check the *levator scapula* (chapter 6), *trapezius* (chapter 3), and *scalene* (chapter 7) muscles, since these can also cause symptoms in the same area. Trigger points in the *rhomboids* will likely only be noticeable when trigger points in these other muscles are inactivated.

Stretches

Trapezius Stretch: See chapter 3 for a stretch that benefits the middle and lower *trapezius*, which will also help treat the *rhomboid* muscles.

Pectoralis Stretch: See chapter 8 for a stretch that relaxes the *pectoralis* muscles, which will also benefit the *rhomboids*.

Exercises

Proper Breathing: See chapter 7, *scalenes* for this exercise.

Also See:
* Levator scapula (chapter 6)
* Trapezius (chapter 3)
* Latissimus dorsi (chapter 13)
* Infraspinatus (chapter 12)
* Pectoralis major (chapter 8)
* Pectoralis minor (chapter 9)

Differential Diagnosis: If you have received a diagnosis of scapulocostal syndrome, be sure to check for trigger points in the rhomboid muscle. You may need to see a chiropractor or osteopathic physician for vertebral misalignments from C_7 to T_5.

Chapter 6: Levator Scapula

This muscle very commonly harbors trigger points, and you may have a stiff neck and an inability to rotate your head.

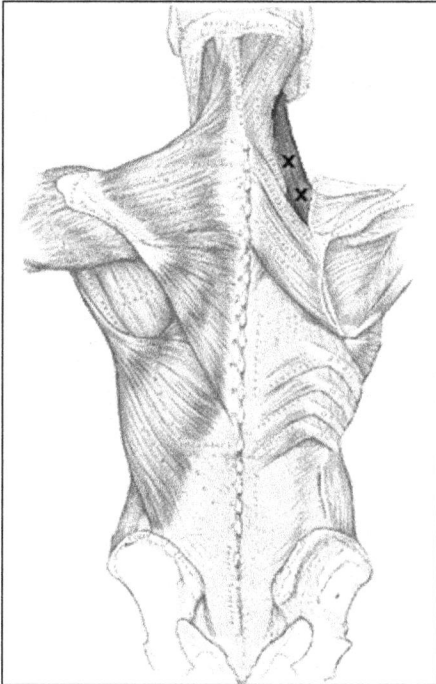

Common Symptoms

- referred pain at the intersection of the neck and shoulders and down the mid-back, and possibly out over the shoulder joint
- limited rotation of the head, so that you have to turn your whole body to look behind you
- pain is more common with movement, but it can also be painful without movement

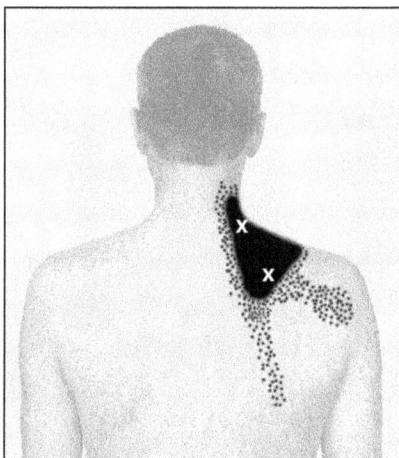

Causes and Perpetuation of Trigger Points

- sitting for long periods of time with your head rotated to one side, as when using a computer screen at the wrong angle or with the copy to the side, or talking to a person sitting next to you
- sitting in a chair with armrests that are too high
- cradling the phone between your shoulder and ear, even with a shoulder cradle
- sleeping with your head at an angle (as when sitting up), tilted with a pillow that is too tall, or tilted on a couch arm, especially when the muscle is fatigued or exposed to a cold draft
- carrying a purse or pack over one shoulder
- swimming using the crawl stroke
- raising your shoulders toward your ears in response to stress, which you may not even realize you are doing
- car accidents
- the initial onset of a cold, flu, or cold sores (oral herpes simplex), even before other viral symptoms become apparent
- walking with a cane that is too high
- trigger points in the *serratus anterior* or upper portion of the *trapezius* (chapter 3)
- imbalances in the lower body such as calf muscle weakness, one leg anatomically shorter than the other, a flattened arch, or a shortened *quadratus lumborum* muscle

This is a list of perpetuating factors specific only to trigger points in <u>this</u> *muscle. For a full list of perpetuating factors that can cause and perpetuate trigger points anywhere in the body and which also apply to this muscle, please see "Appendix A" (found at the end of this book), since some may need to be addressed for lasting pain relief.*

Helpful Hints

- Turn your body or furniture to face the person to whom you are speaking.
- When reading, try to get the music or book at eye level, and make sure your vision does not need correction.
- When using a computer, make sure the monitor is straight ahead and at eye level, and your shoulder rests are at the proper height (your elbows should rest comfortably on the armrests, neither too short so that you lean to one side, nor too tall so that they hike up your shoulders.).
- Use a headset for your phone, and never cradle the phone between your shoulder and ear.
- Don't sleep sitting up or on the couch or an airplane, unless you have head support that will keep your neck as straight as possible.
- Your pillow should be of a height that will keep your spine straight. Chiropractor offices often carry well-designed pillows with cervical support.
- Apply a heating pad or hot pack to your neck, especially at the end of the day.
- Keep cold drafts off of your neck by using a scarf or neck gaiter.
- Notice if you are raising your shoulders toward you head, and relax your shoulders. Keep noticing and relaxing, as you will need to re-train yourself to keep your shoulders

relaxed. Deal with the source of tension, using acupuncture, herbs, homeopathics, and/or counseling.

- Always carry a purse diagonally across your torso, and put the straps of a daypack over both shoulders.
- At the onset of a cold or flu, an acupuncturist will perform cupping or gua sha, which will relax the shoulder muscles and help get rid of the achiness. See the Acute Infections section of "Appendix A" for suggestions on how to minimize the symptoms of acute infections.
- When swimming either vary your stroke, or use a snorkel when doing the crawl stroke.
- Make sure a cane is not so high that it is causing you to hike up a shoulder.

Self-Help Techniques

Applying Pressure

Posterior Neck Pressure: The *posterior neck* pressure will also benefit *levator scapula* trigger points (see chapter 3).

Stretches

Levator Scapula Stretch: Sit on a chair or stool and hook the fingers of one hand around the edge of the seat bottom. Use your other hand to pull your head down to about a 45° angle, or until you feel a gentle stretch; just be sure to feel the stretch on the back of your neck. You may also do this stretch under a hot shower while seated on a stool.

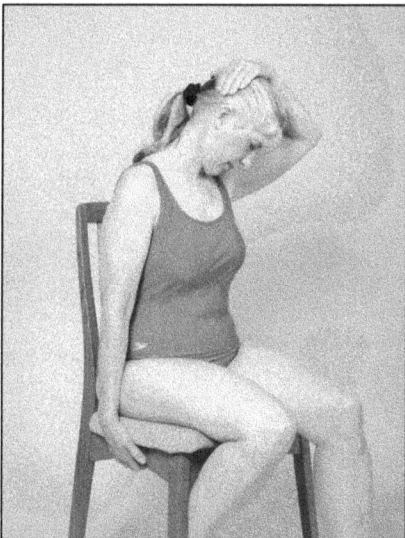

Also See:

*   Scalene (chapter 7)
*   Trapezius (upper portion, chapter 3)

You may also need to check the *posterior neck* and *serratus anterior* muscles, since trigger points in those muscles can either cause similar pain referral patterns or may affect or be affected by *levator scapula* trigger points in some way.

Since trigger points in these muscles don't directly cause shoulder pain, they are not addressed in this book (the posterior neck self-help techniques are found in chapter 3). If you can't relieve your pain with the self-help techniques in this book after six to eight weeks, you may wish to consider whether you need to treat trigger points in these additional muscles, or if you still have perpetuating factors to resolve. Go to the end of this book for other books by the author that provide self-treatment techniques of muscles not covered in this book.

Chapter 7: Scalenes

Scalene trigger points are a major contributor to back, shoulder, and arm pain, and are commonly overlooked. They also contribute to headaches when combined with trigger points in neck and chewing muscles.

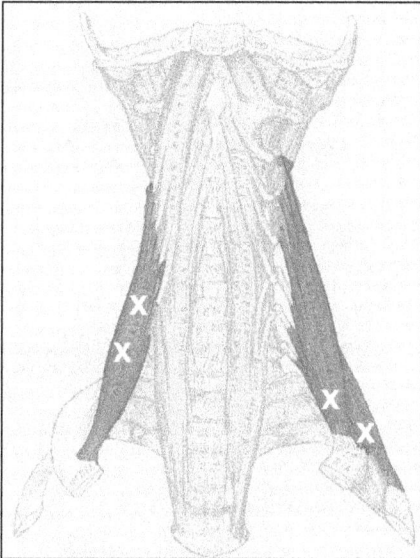

View of front of neck

You may have been diagnosed with **thoracic outlet syndrome**. Thoracic outlet syndrome is a collection of symptoms rather than a specific disease, though it is often stated by health care practitioners as though it was something very specific. There is wide disagreement and confusion in most literature about what symptoms define the condition and what causes it. Some operations successfully treat the symptoms and some do not. Trigger points are frequently overlooked as a cause of abnormal tension in the *scalene* muscles, and are mostly likely a most common cause of thoracic outlet syndrome. It is definitely worth having a trained practitioner check your *scalenes* and the other muscles listed below to see if you may be harboring trigger points, especially if you are considering surgery. Surgery has a less than 50% success rate for thoracic outlet syndrome, most likely because trigger points were not considered or relieved. There may be a few patients with anatomical abnormalities that require surgical correction for complete relief, but the majority of patients will have a higher success rate with non-surgical intervention.

Trigger points in the *pectoralis major* (chapter 8), *latissimus dorsi* (chapter 13), *teres major* (chapter 15), and *subscapularis* (chapter 14) muscles can all refer pain in patterns that mimic thoracic outlet syndrome symptoms. It can be particularly confusing if more than one muscle develops trigger points, so you may need to check all of those muscles. The *trapezius* (chapter 3), *pectoralis minor* (chapter 9), and *levator scapula* (chapter 6) can also refer pain that may be diagnosed as thoracic outlet syndrome. The *subclavius* (chapter 8) muscle can get enlarged and may cause the first rib to be elevated and compress the subclavian vein, so you may need to check for trigger points in that muscle too, and see a chiropractor or osteopathic physician to determine if the first rib needs to be adjusted.

Carpel tunnel syndrome may occur in conjunction with thoracic outlet syndrome, or the symptoms of carpal tunnel syndrome can be mimicked by *scalene* trigger points. If you have been diagnosed with carpel tunnel syndrome, it is worth checking for trigger points in the *scalenes, pectoralis minor (chapter 9)*, and muscles in the forearm.

Common Symptoms

- pain referred to the chest, mid-back, and/or over the outside, back, and front of the arm and into the wrist and hand
- pain that disturbs sleep, but is relieved by sleeping sitting or propped up
- pain on the left side may be mistaken for angina
- perceived numbness of the thumb (but not actual), and tingling
- dropping items unexpectedly
- possibly finger stiffness
- minimal restriction of range-of-motion when rotating your head, but greater restriction when bending it to the side
- you may be able to reproduce pain by turning your head to the side and then putting your chin down toward your shoulder
- you may be able to relieve pain by putting the back of your forearm across your forehead and moving your elbow forward (which moves the collarbone away from the *scalene* muscle)
- a tight *scalene* muscle may elevate the first rib, leading to compressed nerves, arteries, veins, and lymph ducts, causing numbness, tingling, and loss of sensation in the 4th and 5th fingers and side of the hand, and stiffness and swelling in the fingers and back of your hand which is worse in the morning
- phantom limb pain in amputees

Scalenus
anterior
medius
posterior

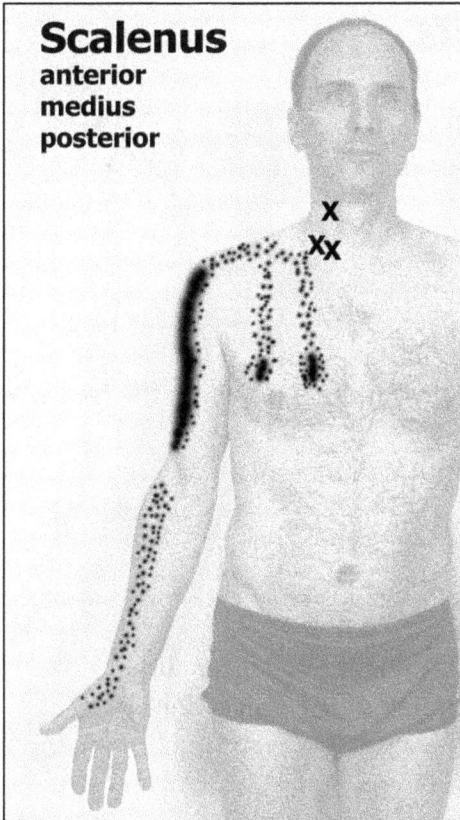

Front referral pattern

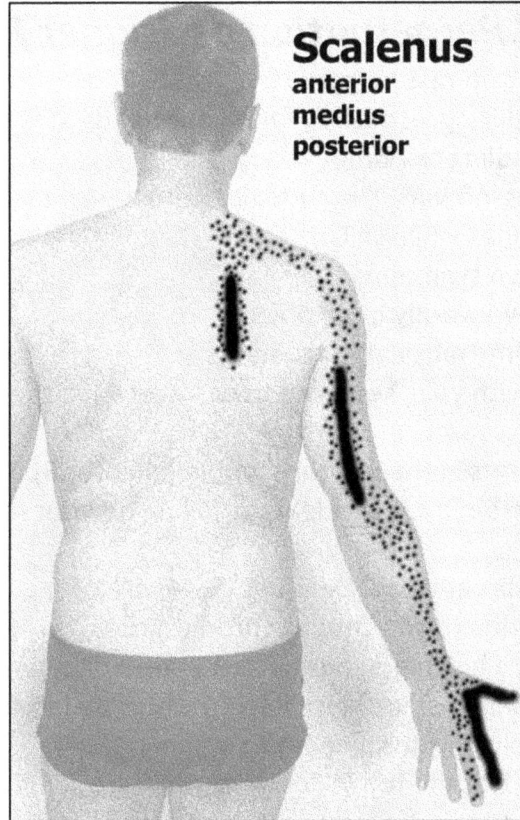

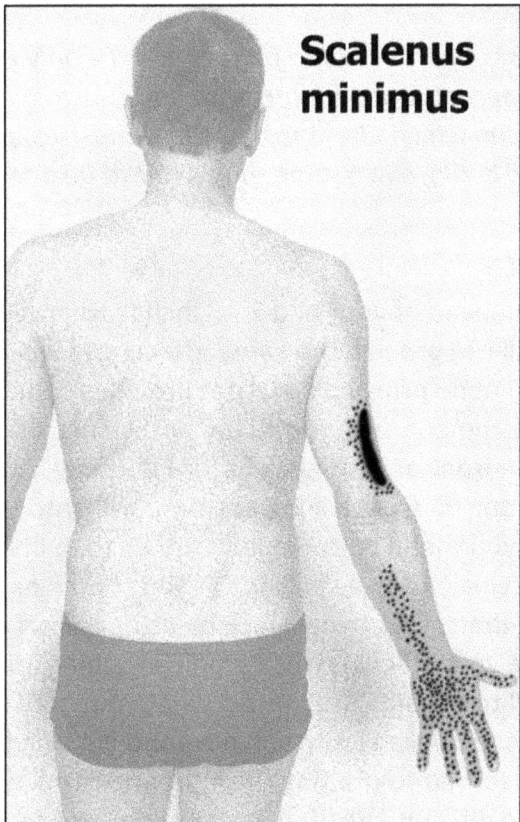

Scalenus
anterior
medius
posterior

Back referral pattern

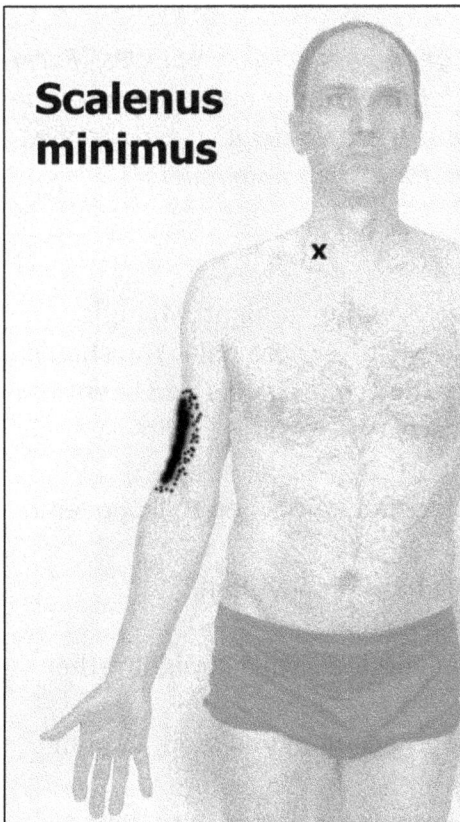

Scalenus minimus

Front referral pattern

Scalenus minimus

Back referral pattern

Causes and Perpetuation of Trigger Points

- improper arm rest height
- pulling or lifting, especially with your hands at waist level
- horse-handling or riding
- playing tug-of-war
- hauling ropes while sailing
- competitive swimming
- carrying awkwardly large objects
- playing some musical instruments
- sleeping with your head and neck lower than the rest of your body, as when the bed is tilted
- trigger points in the *levator scapula* (chapter 6) or *sternocleidomastoid*
- whiplash from a car accident, or falling on your head
- limping
- improper breathing techniques
- coughing due to an acute or chronic illness
- pain from a bulging or herniated cervical disc, which may linger even after surgery
- a shorter leg or small hemipelvis (either the left or right half of the pelvic bone)
- spinal scoliosis (the spine isn't straight)
- an extra rib at the top (a "cervical rib")
- loss of an arm
- surgical removal of a heavy breast

This is a list of perpetuating factors specific only to trigger points in <u>these</u> muscles. For a full list of perpetuating factors that can cause and perpetuate trigger points anywhere in the body and which also apply to these muscles, please see "Appendix A" (found at the end of this book), since some may need to be addressed for lasting pain relief.

Helpful Hints

- Elevate the head of your bed 2 - 3 inches to provide mild traction at night. Multiple pillows will not provide the same effect, and will probably cause more pain. You should get a good non-springy pillow that provides support for the cervical spine and keeps the spine in alignment. A chiropractor's office usually will carry well-designed pillows. Apply heat to the front of your neck before bedtime.
- When getting up from a lying position, roll onto your side first, and when rolling over in bed keep your head on the pillow rather than lifting it.
- Avoid carrying packages in front of your body, or pulling hard on anything.
- Keep cold drafts off of your neck by using a scarf or neck gaiter.
- Make sure your elbow is resting on something, and that you are sitting straight rather than tilted to the side, no matter what your activity.
- When seated, make sure you have good lighting from behind when you read, so your head isn't turned to the side. Don't read in bed.
- If you have difficulty hearing and tend to turn to one side to hear better, turn your entire body to the side, or get a hearing aid if possible.

- Use a headset for the phone, rather than holding it to your ear or cradling it between your ear and shoulder.
- When using a computer, make sure the monitor is straight ahead and at eye level, and your chair arm rests are at the proper height (your elbows and forearms should rest comfortably on the armrests, neither too short so that you lean to one side, nor too tall so that they hike up your shoulders).
- Learn to breathe properly – see the exercise below.
- Eliminate the causes of coughing by treating the underlying illness as quickly as possible (see Perpetuating Factors, Acute or Chronic Infections section of "Appendix A")
- If you have an anatomically short leg or small hemipelvis (even as little as 3/8" or less), you will need to get fitted by a specialist for lifts to compensate, or it is unlikely you will be able to resolve *scalene* trigger points.
- Even if you have an extra "cervical" rib, relieving the *scalene* trigger points may be enough to eliminate symptoms.

Self-Help Techniques

Applying Pressure

I don't teach self-help pressure to this muscle due to all the major nerves and arteries in the front of the neck. You will need to go to a trained practitioner such as a physical therapist or a massage therapist.

Stretches

If you are doing the *pectoralis* stretch (chapter 8), only do the top two positions and not the bottom one until the *scalene* muscles have improved. If you have an extra cervical rib, only do the top position.

Side-Bending Neck Stretch: You may wish to apply heat prior to this stretch. Lie face-up, with the hand of the side you are stretching pinned under your butt.

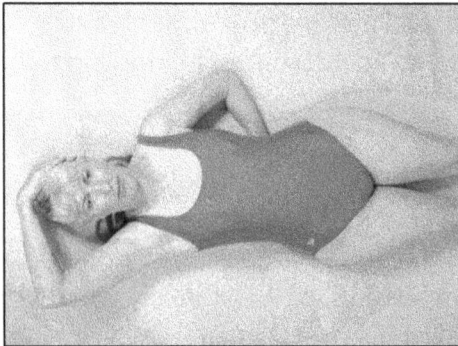

Put your opposite hand over the top of your head and, looking straight at the ceiling, pull your head gently toward your shoulder, then release and take a deep breath.

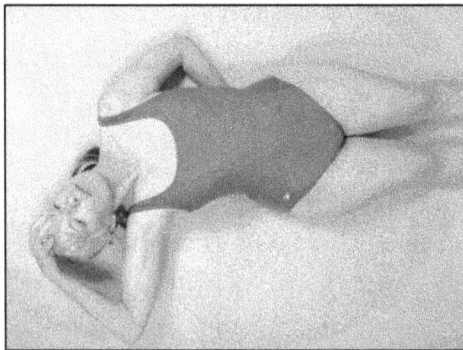

Repeat with your head turned slightly toward the left, and again with your head turned slightly toward the right. This will stretch different parts of the muscle.

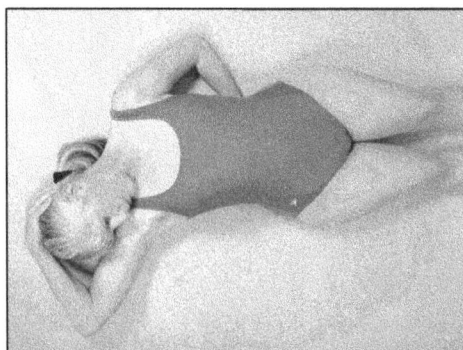

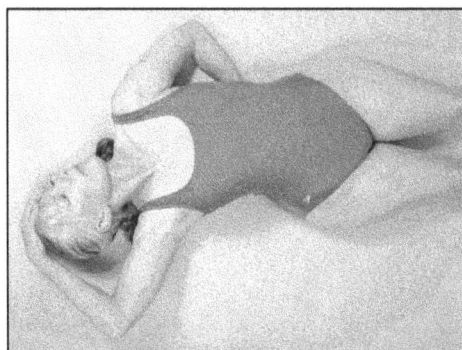

Stretch the opposite side following the same sequence. You may repeat the stretches for each side a few more times.

Scalene Stretch: While sitting up, rotate your head all the way to one side and then bring your chin down. Return to the forward position and take a deep breath. Repeat on the opposite side. You may do this up to four times in each direction.

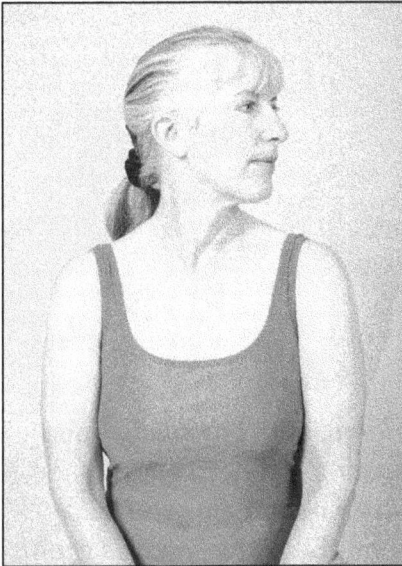

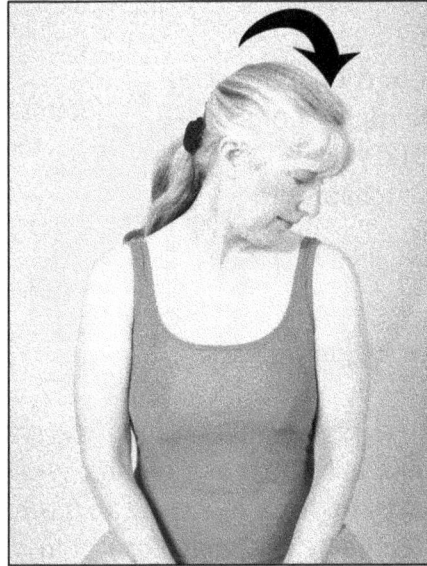

Proper Breathing Exercise: Learning to breathe properly is important for resolving trigger points in several muscles.

Place one hand on your chest and the other on your belly. When you inhale, both hands should rise. As you exhale, both hands should fall. You need to train yourself to notice when you're breathing only into your chest and make sure you start breathing into your belly.

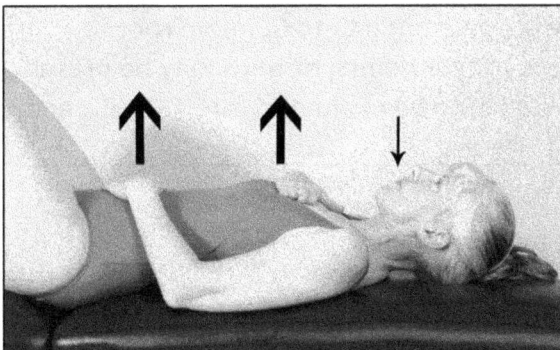

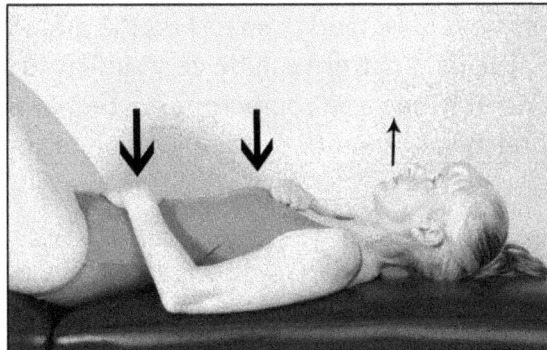

Also See:

*   Levator scapula (chapter 6)
*   Trapezius (chapter 3, upper portion of muscle)
*   Triceps (chapter 18, satellite trigger points)
*   Latissimus dorsi (chapter 13)
*   Pectoralis major / subclavius (chapter 8)
*   Pectoralis minor (chapter 9)
*   Teres major (chapter 15)
*   Subscapularis (chapter 14)
*   Deltoid (chapter 17, satellite trigger points)

You may also need to check the *splenius capitis, sternocleidomastoid, brachialis,* hand extensors (*extensors carpi radialis, extensor carpi ulnaris, and extensor digitorum*) and *brachioradialis,* since trigger points in those muscles can either cause similar pain referral patterns or may affect or be affected by *scalene* trigger points in some way. The *splenius capitis* (posterior neck) pressure and stretches can be found in chapter 3.

Since trigger points in these muscles don't directly cause shoulder pain, they are not addressed in this book. If you can't relieve your pain with the self-help techniques in this book after six to eight weeks, you may wish to consider whether you need to treat trigger points in these additional muscles, or if you still have perpetuating factors to resolve. Go to the end of this book for other books by the author that provide self-treatment techniques of muscles not covered in this book.

Differential Diagnosis: If you are unable to relieve your symptoms with trigger point self-help techniques, you may need to see a health care provider to rule out a C_5 to C_6 nerve root irritation. The pain pattern can be very similar to scalene trigger points, or both may be present. You may need to see a chiropractor or osteopathic physician to be evaluated for T_1, C_4, C_5, and C_6 vertebral misalignments, or for elevation of the first rib.

Chapter 8: Pectoralis Major & Subclavius

This muscle covers much of the chest, and can cause shoulders to be rounded forward in a slumped-looking posture. *Pectoralis major* trigger points can mimic the symptoms of a heart attack, but can also be caused by a heart attack, so heart and lung problems must be ruled out before assuming it is trigger points only.

The *pectoralis major* may get involved in a "frozen shoulder" syndrome. See chapter 2 for a discussion of this condition.

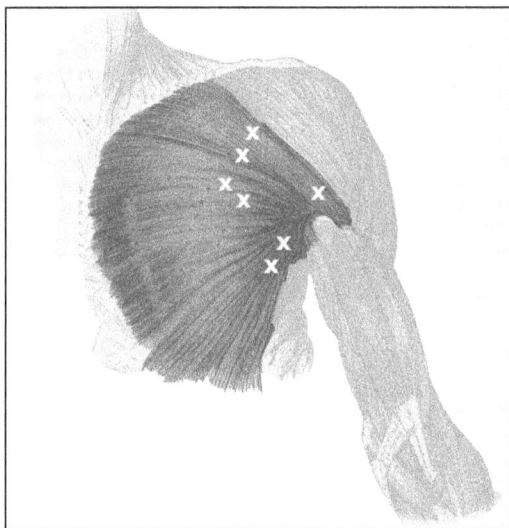

Pectoralis Major muscle, chest area

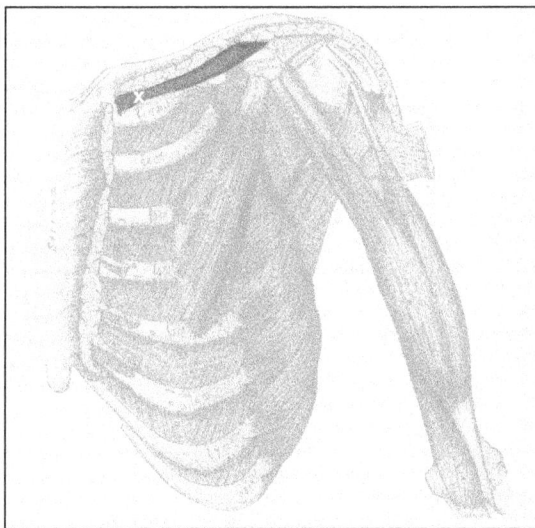

Subclavius muscle, under collarbone

Common Symptoms

- referred pain in the chest, shoulder, breast, and down the inner arm, possibly all the way into the hand
- mid-back pain caused by shortening of the *pectoralis* muscles, even if the *pectoralis* trigger points are latent (not causing referred pain of their own)
- activated or perpetuated trigger points in the *sternocleidomastoid* muscle, along with the subsequent symptoms of those trigger points
- restricted range-of-motion
- chest constriction
- pain may disturb sleep
- breast tenderness, hypersensitivity of the nipple, and/or irritation by clothing on the breast
- there may be a feeling of congestion in the breast, a slight enlargement, and a "doughy" feeling caused by impaired lymph drainage
- a sudden, extreme sharp pain during a sudden overload to the muscle may indicate a torn muscle

Found on right side only

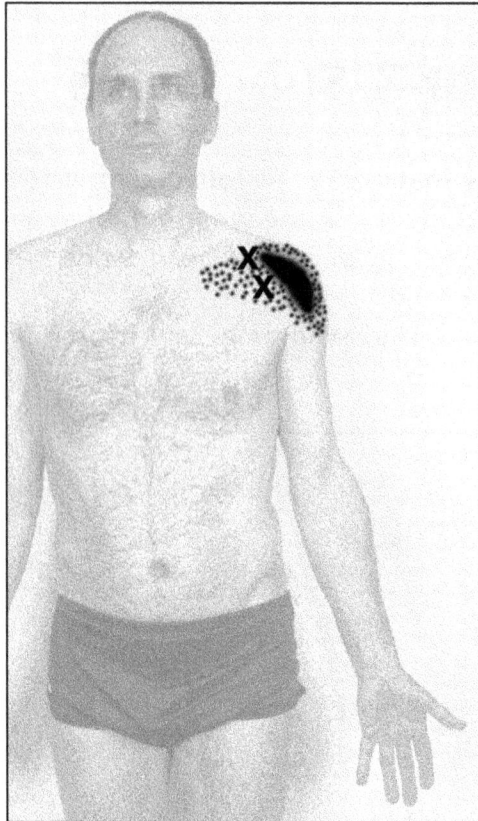

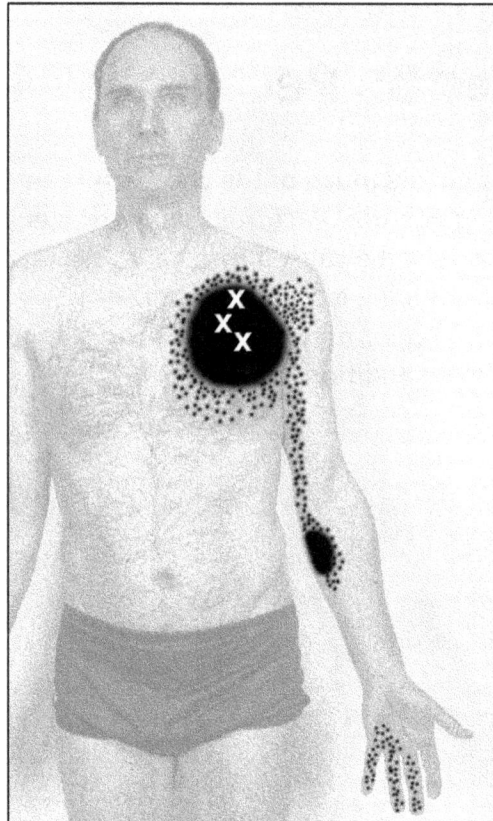

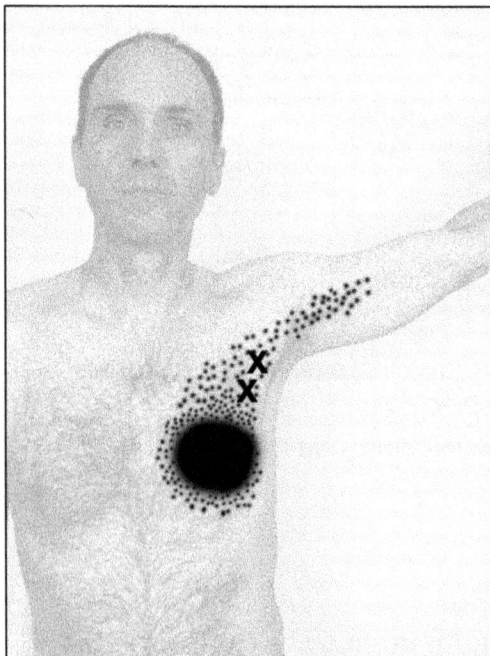

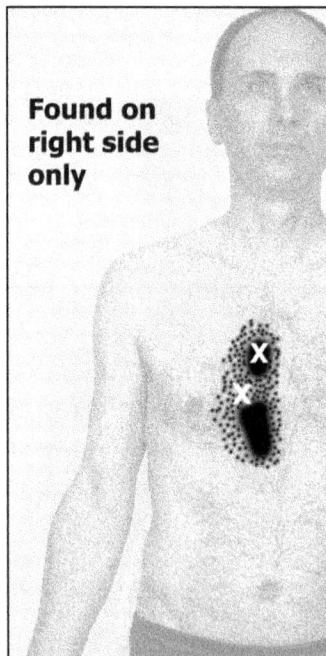

Various pectoralis major referral patterns

- ectopic cardiac arrhythmias such as supraventricular tachycardia, supraventricular premature contractions, or ventricular premature contractions can be caused by a particular point on the right side of the trunk only, between the 5th and 6th rib, about 1-2" to the left of the nipple

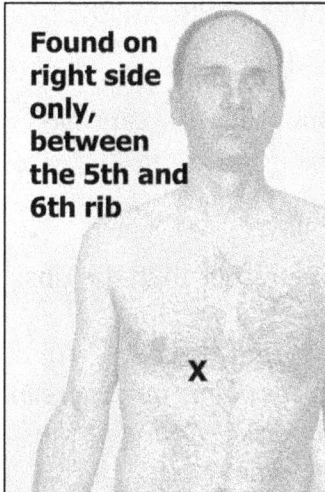

- the *subclavius* can cause pain under the collar bone, down the front upper arm, down the outside of the lower arm, and into the thumb, index, and middle fingers

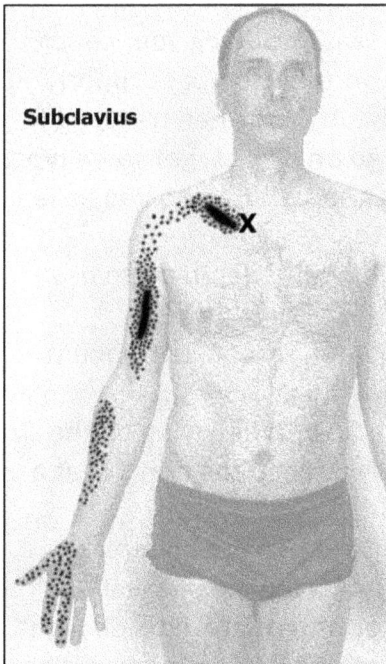

Subclavius front referral pattern   *Subclavius back referral pattern*

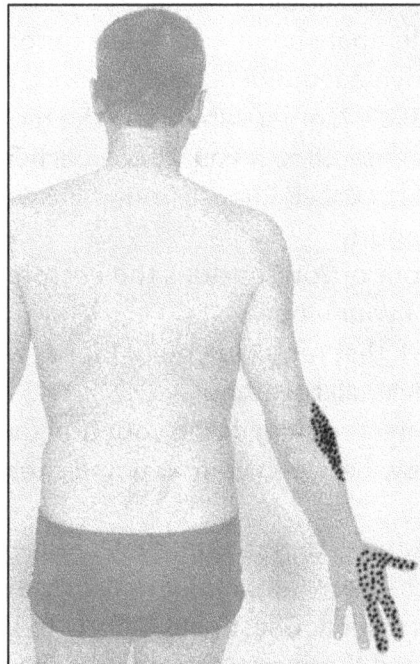

Causes and Perpetuation of Trigger Points

- poor posture while sitting, or slouching while standing, allowing your shoulders to round forward.
- heavy lifting, especially when reaching out
- overuse by bringing your arms together repetitively, as in using a pair of bush clippers
- sustained lifting in front, as with a chainsaw
- your arm being immobilized in a cast or sling
- constant anxiety, probably resulting in holding your breath and subsequently causing trigger points to form
- exposure to cold air when the muscles are fatigued
- a heart attack
- open heart surgery where the incision was through the breastbone rather than the ribs

This is a list of perpetuating factors specific only to trigger points in these muscles. For a full list of perpetuating factors that can cause and perpetuate trigger points anywhere in the body and which also apply to these muscles, please see "Appendix A" (found at the end of this book), since some may need to be addressed for lasting pain relief.

Helpful Hints

- Get a good pair of custom orthotics that will shift your weight slightly to the balls of your feet. This will shift your head back over your shoulders and restore normal cervical and lumbar curves, bring the shoulders back, and open up the chest.
- Get a chair with a good lumbar support. For your car or any seat (including your couch at home) that doesn't have adequate lumbar support, get a portable lumbar support. You may wish to even take a lumbar support to the movie theatre, or when traveling for use on airplanes and in rental cars. If you sit in bleachers or go on picnics, get some type of back support like a **Crazy Creek Chair**™ (found in sporting goods stores) so you have at least some kind of support.
- Crossing your arms in front of you shortens the *pectoralis major* muscle, so try to use armrests at the height of your elbows.
- If you must perform work that requires you to lift or hold tools in front, take frequent breaks, or avoid the activity all together.
- When lying on your unaffected side, drape your arm over a pillow. When lying on the affected side, tuck a pillow between your arm and chest/belly to keep the arm out at a 90-degree angle.
- If your bras leave indentations on the skin, they are too tight and need to be replaced.
- Active trigger points in the *pectoralis major* may cause pain and a feeling of chest constriction that mimics angina. Chest pain is likely to be intermittent and intense with moving the upper arm, and there may also possibly be pain at rest if the trigger points are very active. Pain can disturb sleep. Remember that angina and trigger points can exist concurrently, so you will *still need to undergo cardiac function tests even if you are able to relieve pain with trigger point self-help techniques*. Non-cardiac pain may induce transient T-wave changes in the electrocardiogram, so further tests may be needed. Even with heart disease, pain from trigger points may reflexively diminish the size of the

coronary arteries thereby further increasing myocardial ischemia, so relief of trigger points can increase cardiac circulation in addition to increasing comfort.

- Shortening of the *subclavius* muscle by trigger points can contribute to vascular thoracic outlet syndrome by causing the clavicle to compress the subclavian artery and vein against the first rib.

Self-Help Techniques

Applying Pressure

Pectoralis Pressure: Lie face-down with the arm on the side you are treating next to your side. Place a ball above the breast area and be sure to work all the way out to the armpit. You may need to shift your weight a little to the side you are working on as you work out toward the armpit. You may also try hanging your arm over the side of the bed, if it is high enough to allow your arm to dangle. If you are large-breasted, you may find it easier to place the ball on the end of a couch arm or wall and lean into it, but be sure to keep your arm relaxed.

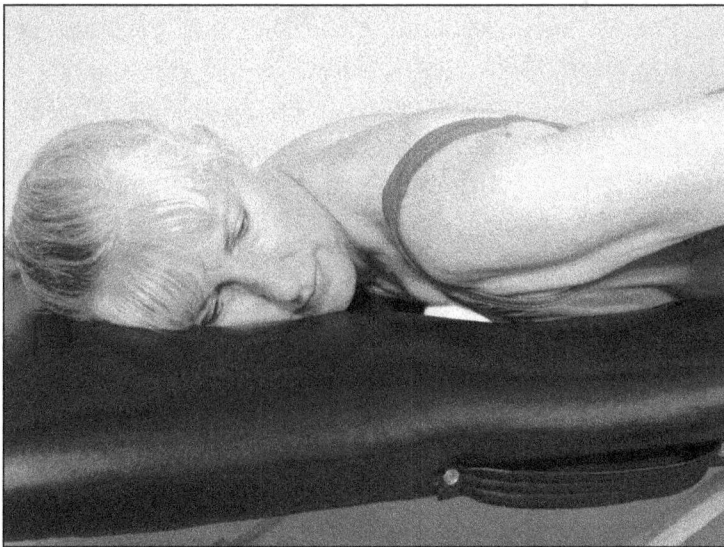

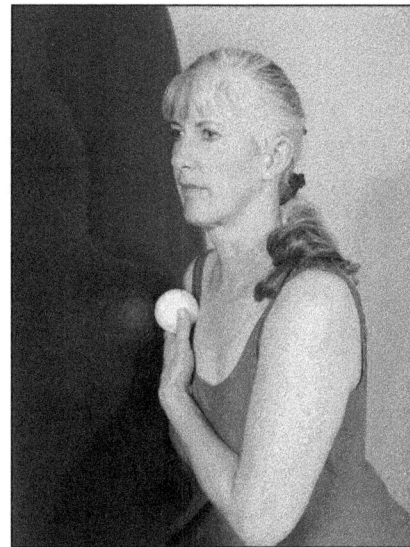

Subclavius Pressure: Much of the *subclavius* muscle is under the collarbone, so you must lean forward, allowing your arm to dangle, which moves the collarbone away from the trunk. With the opposite hand, press under the collarbone with your fingers, especially working closer to the breastbone.

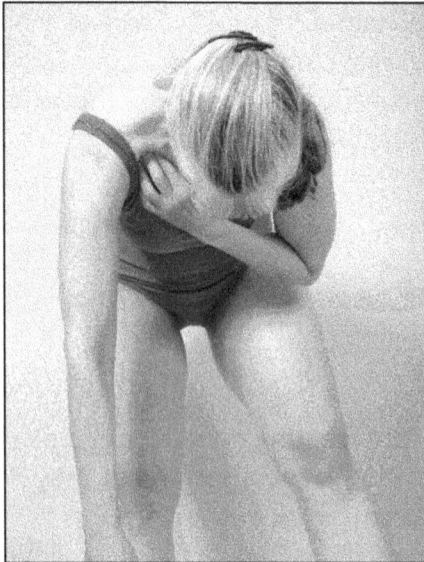

Stretches

Pectoralis Stretch: Stand in a doorway and place your forearm along the door frame, including your elbow, with your upper arm parallel to the floor. With the foot of the same side placed about one step forward, rotate your body gently away from the side you are stretching. Move your forearm up to about a 45° angle and repeat. Bring the forearm down below the first position and repeat. The different forearm positions will stretch different parts of the muscle.

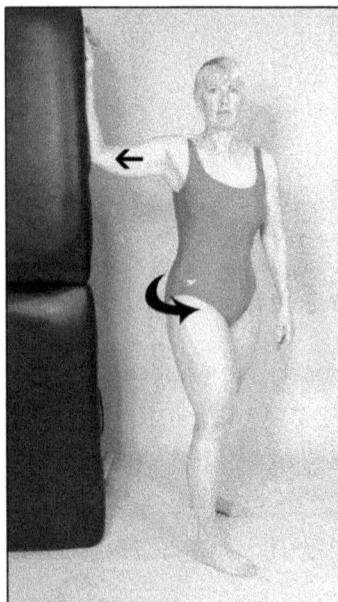

Position 1

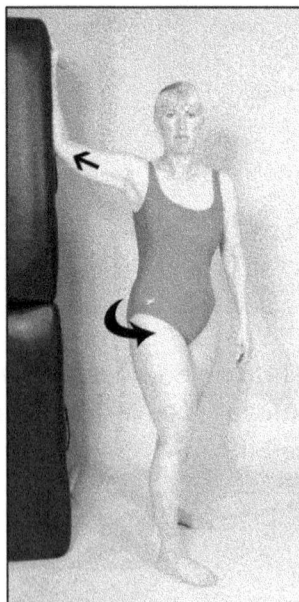

Position 2

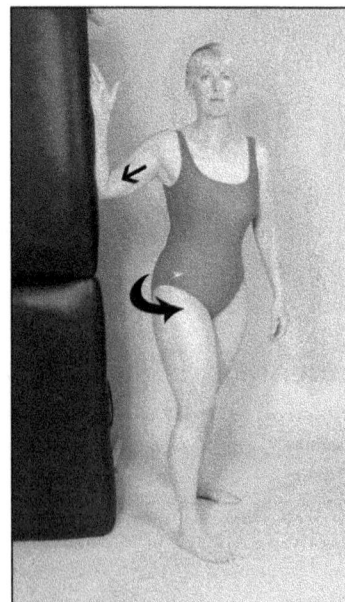

Position 3

Also See:
* Scalene (chapter 7)
* Paraspinal (chapter 4)
* Deltoid (chapter 17, front and rear portions, satellite trigger points)

* Coracobrachialis (chapter 20, satellite trigger points)
* Rhomboid (chapter 5)
* Trapezius (chapter 3)
* Infraspinatus (chapter 12)
* Subscapularis (chapter 14)
* Teres minor (chapter 16)
* Latissimus dorsi (chapter 13)
* Teres major (chapter 15)

If you have a frozen shoulder from pectoralis muscle involvement, you may also need to work on the *subscapularis* (chapter 14), *infraspinatus* (chapter 12), *teres minor* (chapter 16), and posterior *deltoid* (chapter 17) muscles.

If you have been diagnosed with thoracic outlet syndrome, also check the *latissimus dorsi* (chapter 13), *teres major* (chapter 15), *scalenes* (chapter 7), and *subscapularis* (chapter 14) muscles, since trigger points there may mimic thoracic outlet syndrome.

If you have pectoralis major trigger points, you may also need to work on the anterior *deltoid* (chapter 17), *coracobrachialis* (chapter 20), *scalenes* (chapter 7), *trapezius* (chapter 3), and *rhomboid* (chapter 5) muscles, since they will tend to develop satellite trigger points. The *trapezius* and *rhomboid* muscles may become painful after relieving *pectoralis major* trigger points, so you will probably need to perform self-treatment on those muscles after the *pectoralis major* muscle.

You may also need to search for trigger points in the *sternocleidomastoid, sternalis,* and/or *serratus anterior*, since trigger points in those muscles also tend to develop satellite trigger points. Since trigger points in these muscles don't directly cause shoulder pain, they are not addressed in this book. If you can't relieve your pain with the self-help techniques in this book after six to eight weeks, you may wish to consider whether you need to treat trigger points in these additional muscles, or if you still have perpetuating factors to resolve. Go to the end of this book for other books by the author that provide self-treatment techniques of muscles not covered in this book.

Differential Diagnosis: If you are unable to relieve your symptoms with trigger point self-help techniques, you may need to see a health care provider to rule out angina, muscle tears, bicipital tendinitis, supraspinatus tendinitis, subacromial bursitis, medial epicondylitis, lateral epicondylitis, C_5 to C_8 nerve root irritation, intercostal neuritis or radiculopathy, irritation of the bronchi, pleura, or esophagus, a hiatal hernia with reflux, distention of the stomach by gas, mediastinal emphysema, gaseous distention of the splenic flexure of the colon, coronary insufficiency, fibromyalgia, and lung cancer. A sudden, extreme sharp pain during a sudden overload of the muscle may indicate a torn muscle. Skeletal diagnoses that need to be considered include chest wall syndrome, Tietze's syndrome, costochondritis, hypersensitive xiphoid process syndrome, precordial catch syndrome, slipping rib syndrome, and rib-tip syndrome, though many of these may be due either entirely or in part to trigger points.

Chapter 9: Pectoralis Minor

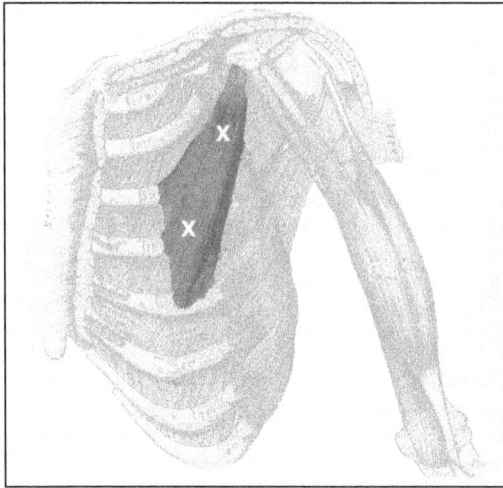

View of front of chest, under pectoralis major muscle

Common Symptoms

- referred pain mainly over the front of the shoulder, and sometimes over the chest and/or down the inside of the arm into the middle, ring, and little fingers
- shoulders that are rounded forward
- range-of-motion restricted when reaching forward and upward, or reaching backward with the arm at shoulder level
- symptoms may mimic angina
- difficulty in taking a deep breath
- a *pectoralis minor* entrapment (pinching the axillary artery and the brachial plexus nerve) can be mis-diagnosed as carpal tunnel syndrome, and will not be resolved by carpal tunnel surgery
- entrapment of the brachial plexus nerve by the *pectoralis minor* muscle causes numbness and uncomfortable sensations of the ring and little fingers, back of the hand, outside of the forearm, and palm side of the thumb, index and middle fingers
- shortening of the *pectoralis minor* muscle fibers as a result of trigger points may lead to "coracoid pressure syndrome," arm pain, and weakness of muscles in the mid-back in the areas of the lower portion of the *trapezius* and *rhomboid* muscles

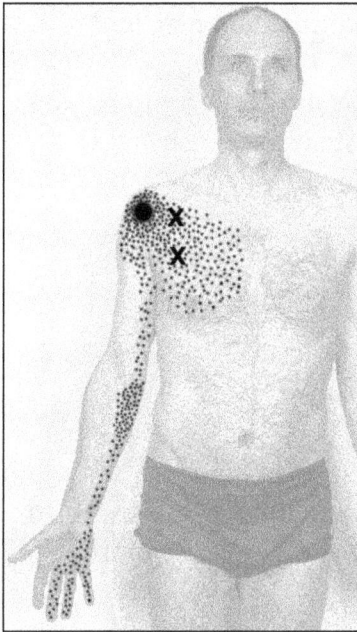

Causes and Perpetuation of Trigger Points

- poor posture, especially when seated
- wearing a daypack or backpack without a chest strap, allowing the shoulder straps to compress the muscle
- gardening
- *scalene* (chapter 7) or *pectoralis major* (chapter 8) trigger points
- weakness of the lower portion of the *trapezius* muscle (chapter 3)
- trauma, such as fractured ribs or firing a rifle with the butt on the chest instead of the front of the shoulder
- using crutches
- coughing and/or improper breathing
- a whiplash injury
- angina pain
- open-heart surgery that was conducted through the breastbone (sternum) rather than the ribs

This is a list of perpetuating factors specific only to trigger points in <u>this</u> muscle. For a full list of perpetuating factors that can cause and perpetuate trigger points anywhere in the body and which also apply to this muscle, please see "Appendix A" (found at the end of this book), since some may need to be addressed for lasting pain relief.

Helpful Hints

- Modify or replace your mis-fitting furniture. Your knees should fit under your desk, and the chair needs to be close enough that you can lean against your backrest. Your elbows should rest on either your work surface or armrests at the same height. Your elbows and forearms should rest evenly on the armrests. Your computer screen should be directly in front of you, and the copy attached to the side of the screen, so that you may look directly forward as much as possible.

- Use crutches properly by supporting your weight on your hands, not your armpits.
- Be sure to use a pack with proper shoulder padding and a chest strap to distribute weight away from the armpit area.
- Learn to breathe properly; see chapter 7.
- Avoid bras that compress the *pectoralis minor* muscle. Try to find one with a wider shoulder strap or a padded strap.

Self-Help Techniques

Check for trigger points in the *pectoralis major* (chapter 8) and *scalene* (chapter 7) muscles, since they will keep trigger points in the *pectoralis minor* activated. You may need to check the *deltoid* (chapter 17) for satellite trigger points after treating the *pectoralis* muscles.

Applying Pressure

Pectoralis Major Pressure: The *pectoralis major* pressure (chapter 8) will also treat the underlying *pectoralis minor* muscle.

Stretches

Pectoralis Stretch: See chapter 8.

Also See:
* Pectoralis major (chapter 8)
* Scalene (chapter 7)
* Deltoid (chapter 17, anterior portion, satellite trigger points)

You may also need to search for trigger points in the *sternalis* and *sternocleidomastoid*, since trigger points in these muscles may be involved. Since trigger points in these muscles don't directly cause shoulder pain, they are not addressed in this book. If you can't relieve your pain with the self-help techniques in this book after six to eight weeks, you may wish to consider whether you need to treat trigger points in these additional muscles, or if you still have perpetuating factors to resolve. Go to the end of this book for other books by the author that provide self-treatment techniques of muscles not covered in this book.

Differential Diagnosis: If you are unable to relieve your symptoms with trigger point self-help techniques, you may need to see a health care provider to rule out *true* thoracic outlet syndrome, C_7 and C_8 nerve root irritation, supraspinatus tendonitis, bicipital tendonitis, and medial epicondylitis. You may need to see a chiropractor or osteopathic physician to be evaluated for elevation of the third, fourth, and fifth ribs.

Chapter 10: Serratus Posterior Superior

This muscle frequently contains trigger points, and often gets missed by therapists because the shoulder blade needs to be moved out of the way in order to access the most common trigger point. Placing the arm over the side of the massage table moves the shoulder blade forward and exposes the trigger point.

Common Symptoms

- referred pain over the shoulder blade (often a deep ache), down the back of the arm and into the little finger
- occasionally pain may be felt in the upper chest area
- pain may be increased by lifting objects out in front of you
- pain may be increased by lying on the affected side, due to the shoulder blade pressing on the trigger points
- referred numbness into the hand

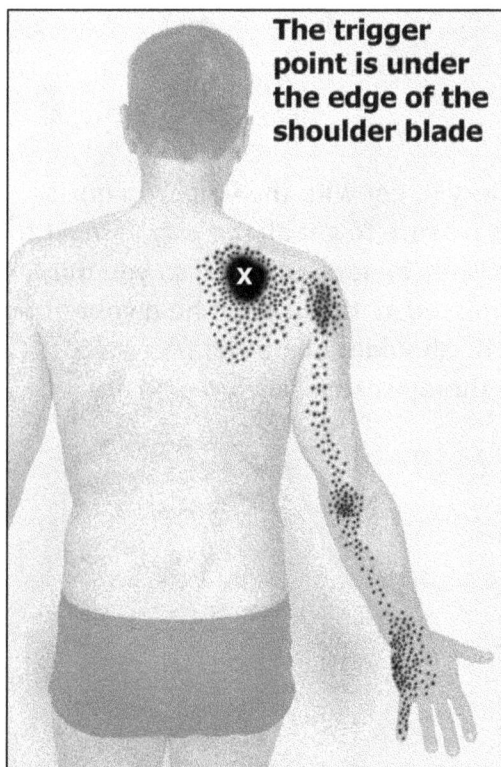

The trigger point is under the edge of the shoulder blade

Back referral pattern   *Front referral pattern*

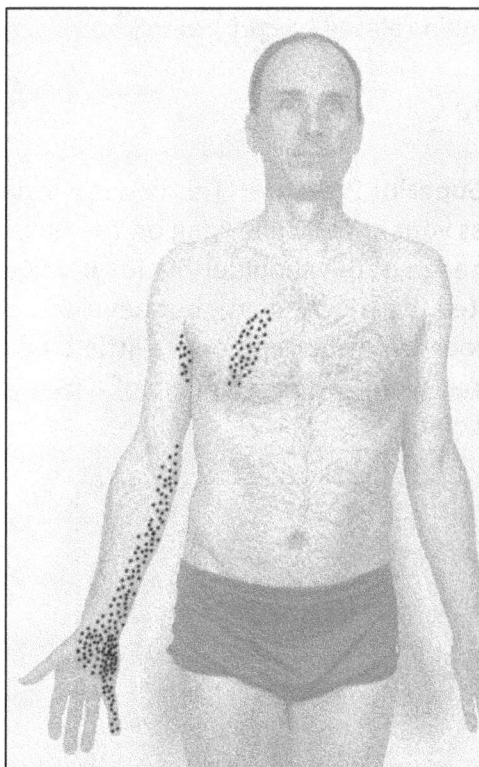

Causes and Perpetuation of Trigger Points

- writing at a high desk or table
- reaching far forward frequently
- the shoulder blade compressing the muscle against the underlying rib

- coughing, asthma, emphysema, and improper breathing techniques
- severe scoliosis

This is a list of perpetuating factors specific only to trigger points in <u>this</u> muscle. For a full list of perpetuating factors that can cause and perpetuate trigger points anywhere in the body and which also apply to this muscle, please see "Appendix A" (found at the end of this book), since some may need to be addressed for lasting pain relief.

Helpful Hints
- Use a lumbar support at work, home, and while traveling.
- Learn to breathe properly (see *scalenes*, chapter 7).

Self-Help Techniques

Also check the *scalene* muscles (chapter 7), since trigger points in those muscles may cause trigger points in the *serratus posterior superior*, or occasionally vice versa. The *rhomboid* muscle (chapter 5) and the *iliocostalis thoracis, longissimus thoracis, and multifidi* muscles (chapter 4) may contain related trigger points.

Applying Pressure

Serratus Posterior Superior Pressure: This one is a little tricky to get with the ball. You *must* hold your arm across your chest while lying on the ball, and be sure to get all the way up next to the top of the inner edge of the shoulder blade. It will also likely be tender lower, so you may think you have treated the trigger point, but have actually missed it. If you don't hold your arm across your chest, your arm will drop down a little bit and the shoulder blade will cover the trigger point. You may want to seek the help of a massage therapist to make sure you are finding this trigger point.

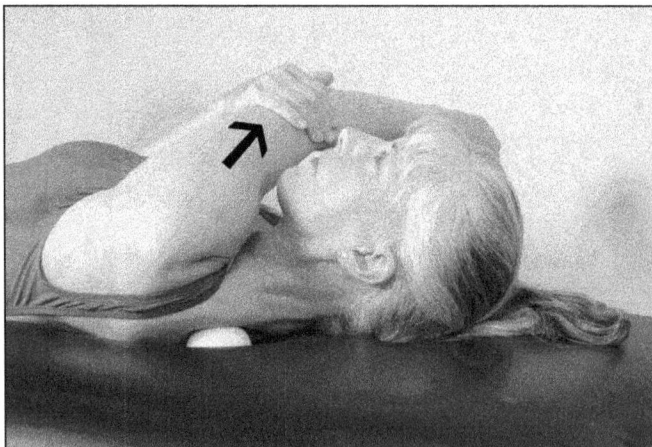

Exercises

Proper Breathing: See chapter 7, *scalenes* for this exercise.

Also See:
* Scalene (chapter 7)
* Rhomboid (chapter 5)
* Paraspinal (chapter 4)

Differential Diagnosis: If you are unable to relieve your symptoms with trigger point self-help techniques, you may need to see a health care provider to be evaluated for thoracic outlet syndrome, a C_7/C_8 nerve root irritation, olecranon bursitis, and ulnar neuropathy. Referred numbness from serratus posterior superior trigger points into the C_8/T_1 distribution of the hand may be mistaken for a nerve root irritation, so be sure to check for trigger points if you have been given this diagnosis. You may need to see a chiropractor or osteopathic physician for evaluation of a T_1 vertebra out of alignment. There will usually be tenderness over the vertebrae if this is the case.

Chapter 11: Supraspinatus

This is one of the muscles forming the "rotator cuff," along with the *infraspinatus* (chapter 12), *teres minor* (chapter 16), and *subscapularis* (chapter 14).

See chapter 2 for more information on "rotator cuff injuries." Pain is more often due to trigger points, and may also be present even if a tear is confirmed, especially if tightness in the muscle from trigger points contributed to the overload that lead to the tear.

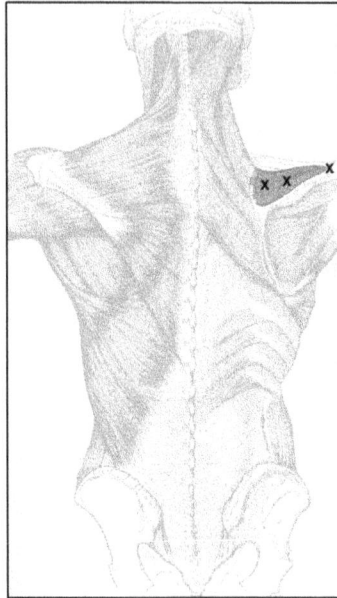

View of back of trunk   *Back view of left shoulder blade*

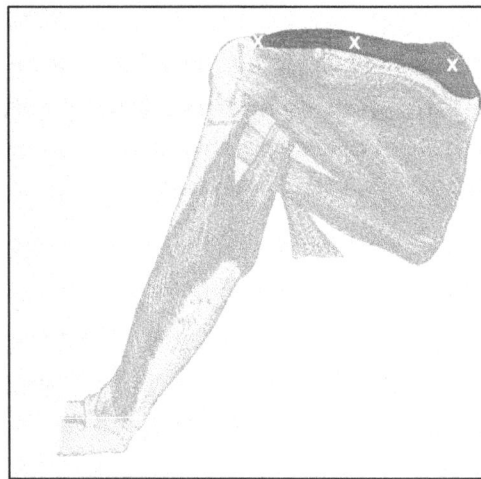

Common Symptoms

- a deep ache in the shoulder area, mainly around the outside of the upper end of the upper arm, and it may be felt strongly in the elbow, and/or run down the outside of the arm, sometimes all the way to the wrist
- pain is worse with lifting the arm, and there is a dull ache when resting the arm
- the shoulder may make clicking or snapping sounds, probably due to the tight muscle interfering with the normal glide of the shoulder joint
- moderately restricted range-of-motion is more noticeable when reaching toward your head or with sports
- pain may get mis-diagnosed as subdeltoid bursitis, though both may be present
- possibly stiffness and aching when in bed
- an inability to reach behind your back and touch the opposite shoulder blade with your fingers

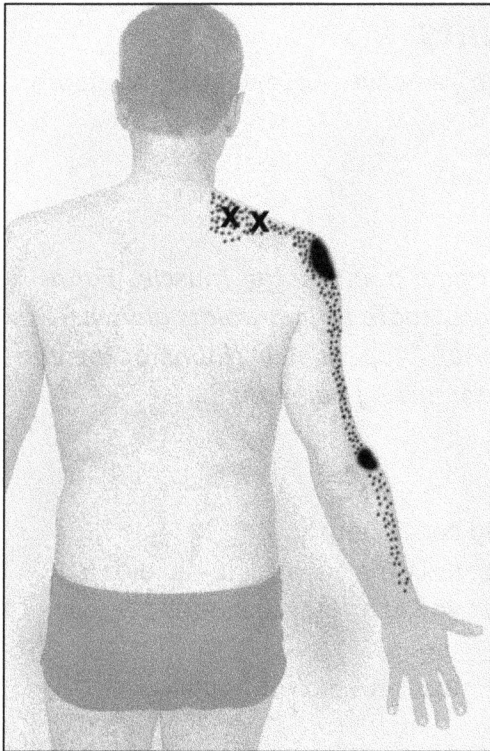

Back referral pattern

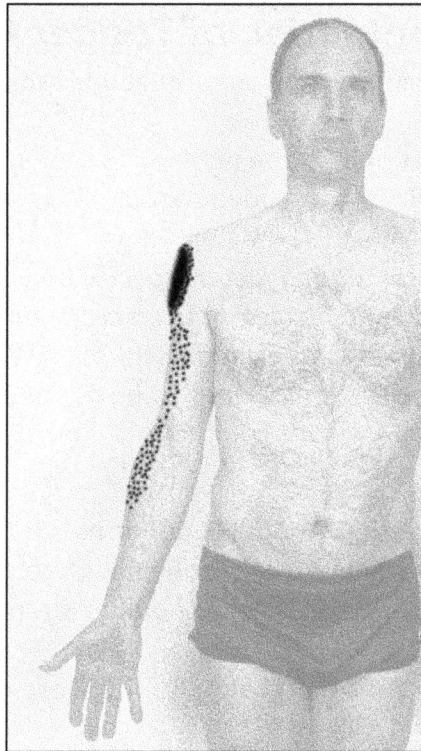

Front referral pattern

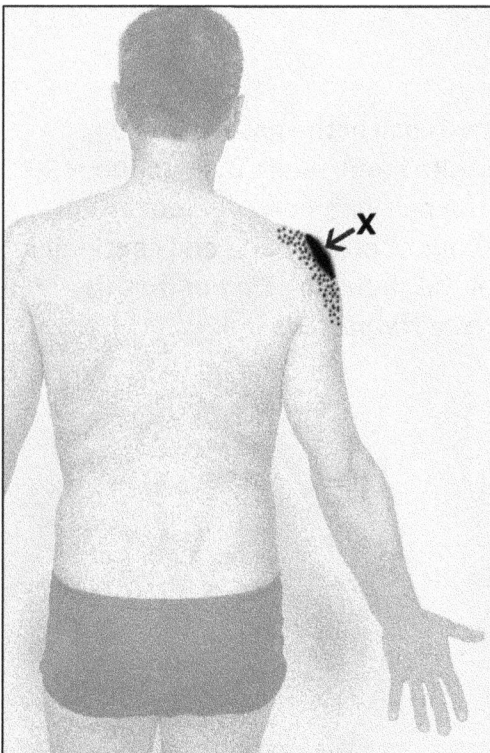

Back referral pattern, supraspinatus attachment found in joint space

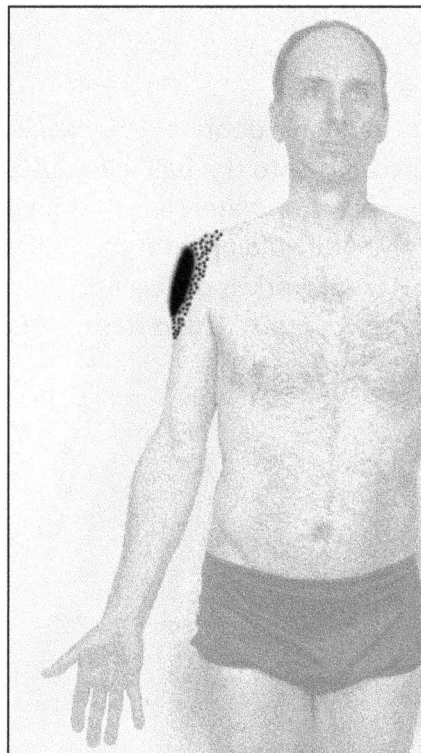

Front referral pattern, supraspinatus attachment

Causes and Perpetuation of Trigger Points

- carrying heavy objects with your arm at your side (i.e., a heavy purse, laptop, briefcase, or luggage)
- walking a dog that pulls at the leash
- lifting a heavy object to or above shoulder height

This is a list of perpetuating factors specific only to trigger points in <u>this</u> muscle. For a full list of perpetuating factors that can cause and perpetuate trigger points anywhere in the body and which also apply to this muscle, please see "Appendix A" (found at the end of this book), since some may need to be addressed for lasting pain relief.

Helpful Hints

- Don't lift items overhead or hold your arms out or up continuously.
- Get luggage with wheels or ask for help with carrying it. Use a daypack instead of a briefcase or heavy purse, or get a shoulder strap that you can wear diagonally across your torso.
- Get a head halter for a dog that pulls. It will prevent most breeds from pulling.

Self-Help Techniques

Applying Pressure

Supraspinatus Pressure: Stand in a doorway and place a tennis ball in the groove in the doorjamb, and continue to hold onto the ball with your opposite hand. Bend over at about 90° *and be sure to let your head go completely limp!* Lean into the ball with however much pressure you want to apply. Still holding onto the ball with your opposite hand and continuing to keep your head fully relaxed, work spots across the top of the shoulder. **Do not do this technique if you have neck problems. Use a Backnobber© (see chapter 3).**

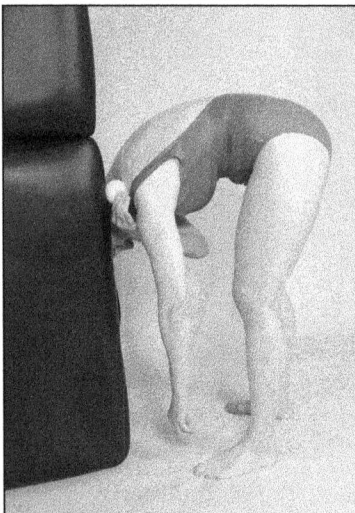

Stretches

Infraspinatus Stretch. The *infraspinatus* stretch (chapter 12) will also benefit the *supraspinatus*. If there is any suspicion of a tear in one of the rotator cuff muscles, *do not stretch this muscle until a tear is ruled out by an MRI, arthrogram, or ultrasound. Prior to getting one of these tests, or if a tear is confirmed, only do the pressure technique above.*

Also See:
*   Trapezius (chapter 3)
*   Infraspinatus (chapter 12)
*   Latissimus dorsi (chapter 13)
*   Deltoid (chapter 17, satellite trigger points)
*   Subscapularis (chapter 14)
*   Teres minor (chapter 16)

Differential Diagnosis: If you are unable to relieve your symptoms with trigger point self-help techniques, you may need to see a health care provider to rule out cervical arthritis or spurs with nerve root irritation, entrapment of the suprascapular nerve, or a brachial plexus injury. Subdeltoid bursitis, rotator cuff tears, and supraspinatus trigger points may all cause tenderness where the tendons of the rotator cuff muscles attach at the shoulder joint, but only trigger points will cause spot tenderness in the mid portion of the supraspinatus muscle. A rotator cuff tear causes severe pain and usually exhibits a limited arc of motion, and must be diagnosed by an MRI, arthrogram, or ultrasound. You may need to see a chiropractor or osteopathic physician to be evaluated for a C_5 or C_6 vertebra out of alignment.

Chapter 12: Infraspinatus

One of the four muscles forming the "rotator cuff," the *infraspinatus* muscle lies over the back of the shoulder blade, or scapula. Trigger points in this area are becoming increasingly common as people spend more time on computers, especially on the side used as the "mouse arm."

The other three muscles comprising the rotator cuff are the *supraspinatus* (chapter 11), *teres minor* (chapter 16), and *subscapularis* (chapter 14). See chapter 2 for more information on "rotator cuff injuries." Pain is more often due to trigger points, and may also be present even if a tear is confirmed, especially if tightness in the muscle from trigger points contributed to the overload that lead to the tear.

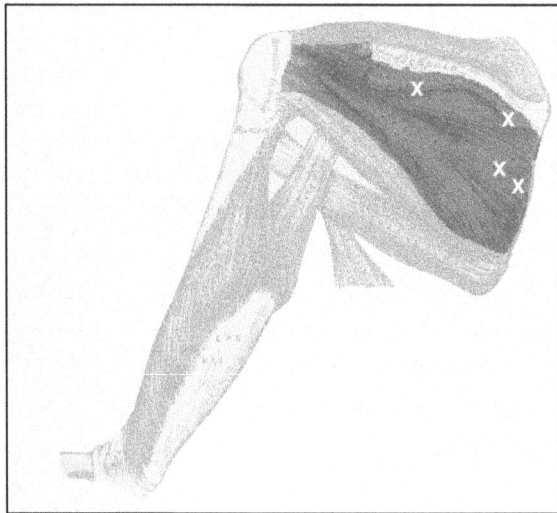

Back view of left shoulder blade

Common Symptoms

- deep pain on the front of the shoulder and deep within the joint, and sometimes into the forearm and occasionally the fingers or into the base of the skull
- occasionally pain will refer to the mid-back area over the *rhomboid* muscles (chapter 5), and sometimes this will activate and perpetuate the lower *trapezius* trigger points (chapter 7), which must be inactivated before *infraspinatus* trigger points can be inactivated
- possibly referred pain when sleeping on either the affected or opposite side at night thereby disrupting sleep
- the arm may "fall asleep" at night, and sometimes even during the day
- difficulty reaching behind your back or sometimes raising your arm to your head in front
- shoulder girdle fatigue
- "weakness" of grip
- loss of mobility
- hyperhydrosis in the area of pain referral (excessive sweating at times that you would not normally sweat, i.e., not due to exercising or extreme heat)

- lack of power with tennis strokes
- entrapment of the suprascapular nerve can cause shoulder pain and atrophy of the *infraspinatus* muscle

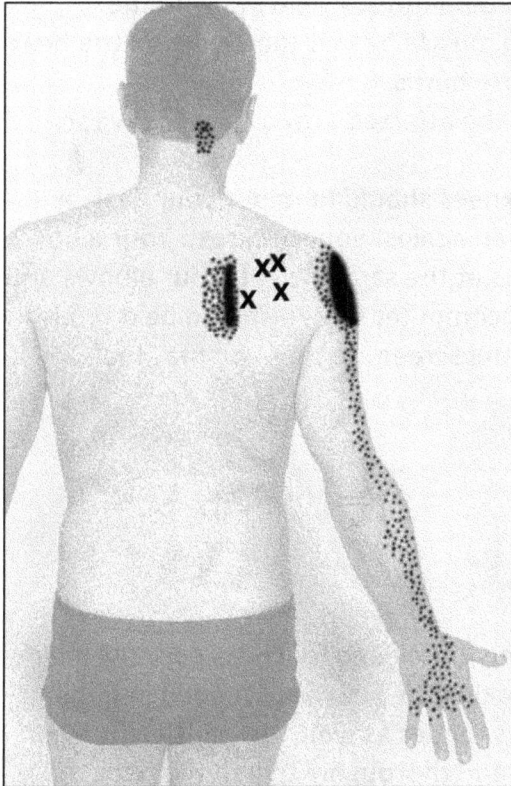

Back referral pattern   *Front referral pattern*

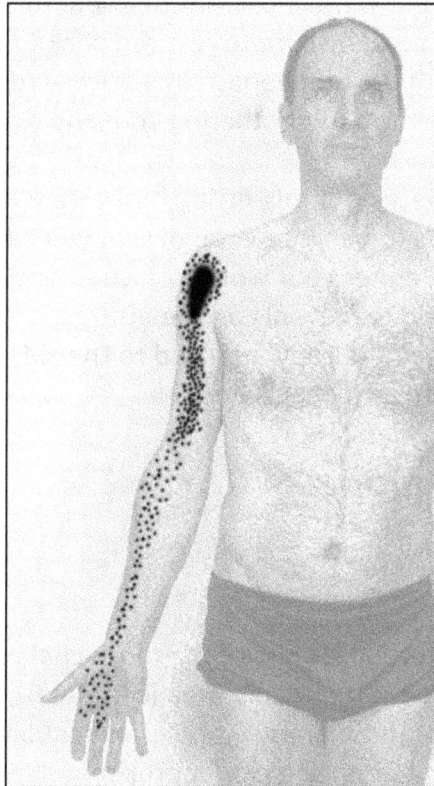

Causes and Perpetuation of Trigger Points
- pulling a sled, wagon, or person behind you
- reaching behind you to get something off a night stand
- hard tennis serves
- pushing yourself with ski poles
- a sudden overload of the muscle by arresting yourself from a fall, or trying to hold onto something heavy
- anything that requires you to hold your arms out in front of you for extended periods of time with your arms not well supported, such as computer use (especially your "mouse arm"), kayaking, driving, or tennis

This is a list of perpetuating factors specific only to trigger points in <u>this</u> *muscle. For a full list of perpetuating factors that can cause and perpetuate trigger points anywhere in the body and which also apply to this muscle, please see "Appendix A" (found at the end of this book), since some may need to be addressed for lasting pain relief.*

Helpful Hints

- Avoid activities that overload the muscles, such as holding your arms over your head while styling your hair, or reaching backward to reach items on a bedside table.
- Apply heat packs to the muscle at bedtime for 15-20 minutes. As always with the application of heat, be sure to rest the pack on the muscle, rather than lying on the heat pack, which can cut off needed circulation and cause burns.
- Lie on the side that isn't bothering you, and drape the affected arm over a pillow for support.
- Modify or replace your mis-fitting furniture. Your knees should fit under your desk, and the chair needs to be close enough that you can lean against your backrest. Your elbows should rest on either your work surface or armrests at the same height. Your elbows and forearms should rest evenly on the armrests. Your computer screen should be directly in front of you, and the copy attached to the side of the screen, so that you may look directly forward as much as possible.

Self-Help Techniques

Applying Pressure

Infraspinatus Pressure: This is one of the more challenging muscles to teach, as patients nearly always initially work in the *rhomboid* area (chapter 5), thinking they have succeeded in finding the *infraspinatus* since the *rhomboid* area is almost always tender as well. Lie on the affected side, with your arm out at an angle of approximately 90°, and thoroughly search the back of your shoulder blade. If you are lying on your back, you are probably getting too far in toward the spine. I find it is helpful to have the patient reach under their arm and locate the muscle with their fingertips first, as with most people this is where their fingers will reach. Be sure to work all the way out to the armpit and then you will know you are treating the correct area. Most people will need to do this on the bed with a fairly soft ball, since this muscle is usually quite tender.

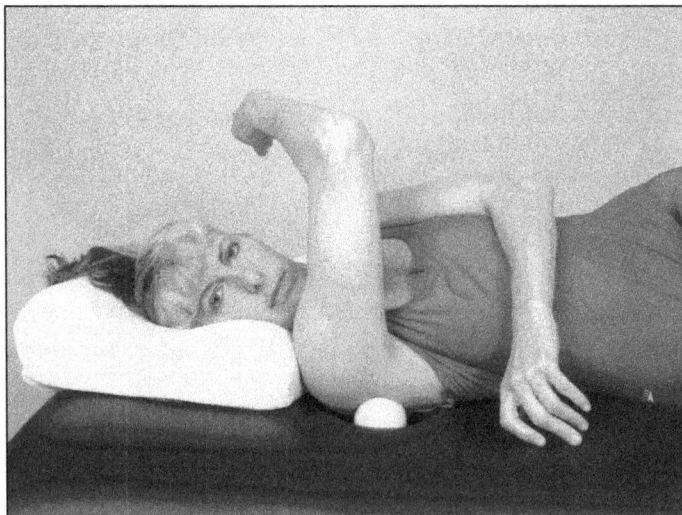

If lying on the affected side is too painful, an alternative is to put a ball in a long sock, dangle the sock over your shoulder, and lean against a wall or couch with however much pressure is comfortable. Remember you will need to angle your body out a little bit from the wall or couch, otherwise you will get in too close to the spine and miss the *infraspinatus* muscle. The affected arm should be totally relaxed. When the tenderness decreases, start performing your self-treatment on the bed, since this is the preferred position.

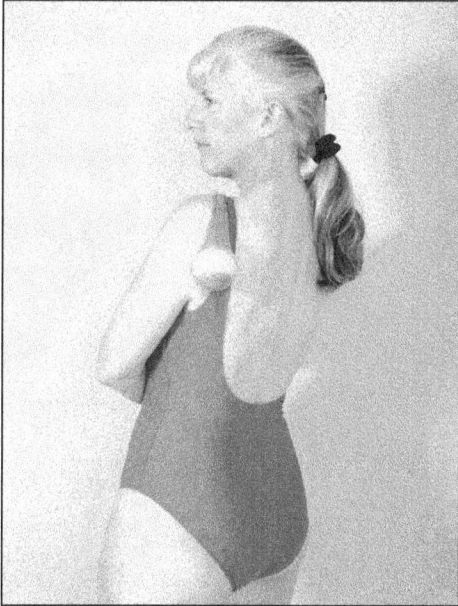

Area to work on with ball

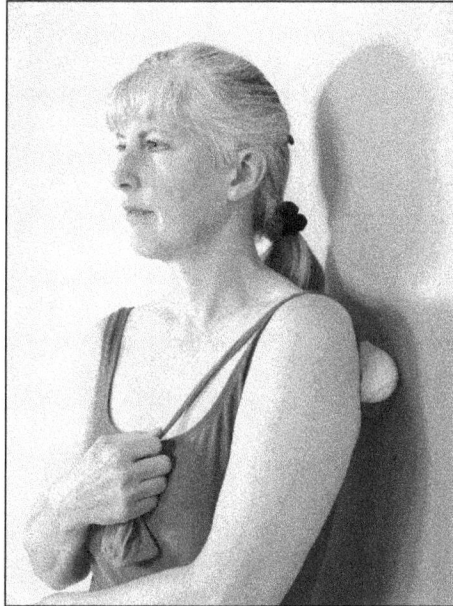

Stretches

Infraspinatus Stretch: Stretch by grasping the affected arm above the elbow and bring your arm across your chest.

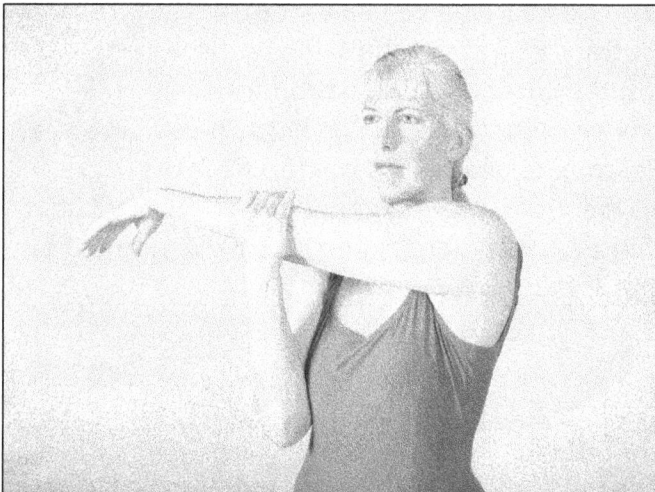

Then put your affected arm behind your back, use the opposite hand to grasp at the wrist, and gently pull on the arm. You can do this in a shower to help facilitate the stretch.

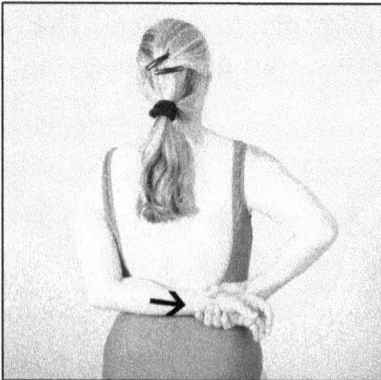

Also See:

* Supraspinatus (chapter 11)
* Latissimus dorsi (chapter 13)
* Teres major (chapter 15)
* Teres minor (chapter 16)
* Deltoid (chapter 17)
* Biceps (chapter 19)
* Pectoralis major (chapter 8)
* Subscapularis (chapter 14)

Differential Diagnosis: If you are unable to relieve your symptoms with trigger point self-help techniques, you may need to see a health care provider to rule out entrapment of the suprascapular nerve at the spinoglenoid notch where it passes from the supraspinatus to the infraspinatus muscle. This can be diagnosed by a test for prolonged nerve conduction latency and/or atrophy of the infraspinatus, and the abnormality causing it confirmed by an MRI or ultrasound. Arthritis in the shoulder joint can also cause a similar pain pattern.

Since infraspinatus trigger point pain referral patterns are the same as those of C_5, C_6, and C_7 nerve root irritation due to disc problems, the latter needs to be confirmed by considering additional neurological problems and electromyographic findings. If you have been unsuccessfully treated for bicipital tendonitis or scapulohumeral syndrome, check the infraspinatus, biceps, pectoralis major, and pectoralis minor for trigger points. A rotator cuff tear causes severe pain and usually exhibits a limited arc of motion, and must be confirmed by an MRI, arthrogram, or ultrasound.

Chapter 13: Latissimus Dorsi

The *latissimus dorsi* muscle is an often-overlooked source of trigger point referral, primarily because there are many other muscles that cause symptom referral in the same area. If you have pain in this area and working on other muscles has given none or only temporary relief, be sure to check this muscle for tenderness. The trigger point under the armpit is the more common culprit.

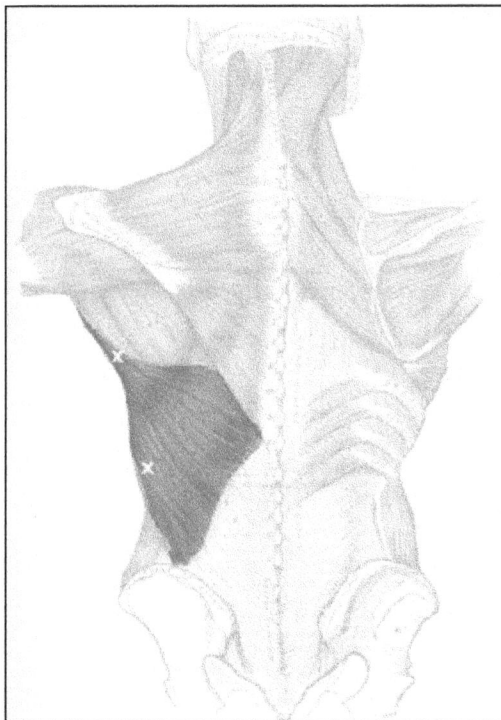

Back view of trunk

Common Symptoms

- the main area of symptom referral is under and adjacent to the bottom of the shoulder blade, with a constant, dull ache
- pain can sometimes travel down the arm and into the ring and little fingers
- there is a less common trigger point on the side above the waist that refers pain to the front of the shoulder and sometimes just above the hip area
- it is difficult to obtain relief by moving around, and pain will be worse as you reach up and out with a heavy object in your hands
- initially pain may *only* be caused by lifting a heavy object in front of you, and not felt at rest
- an inability to identify any particular activity that aggravates mid-back pain

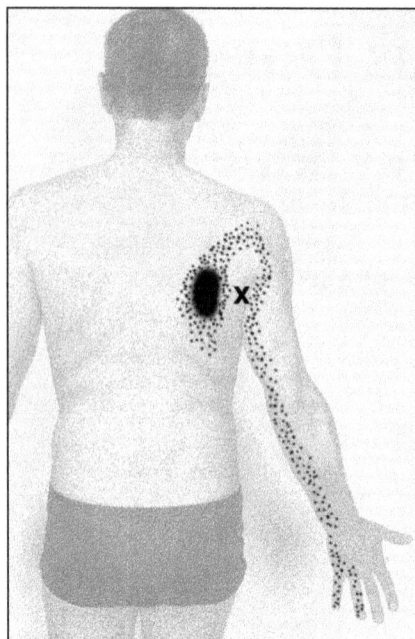

Back referral pattern   **Front referral pattern**   **Side referral pattern**

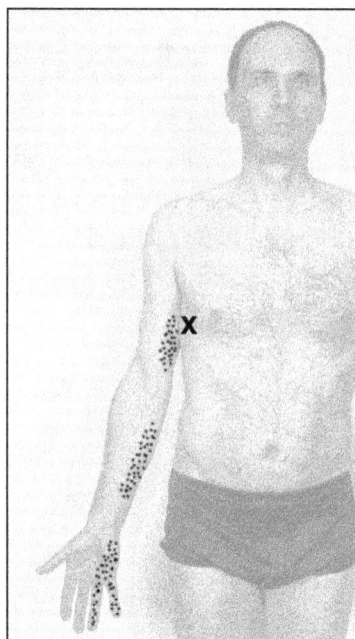

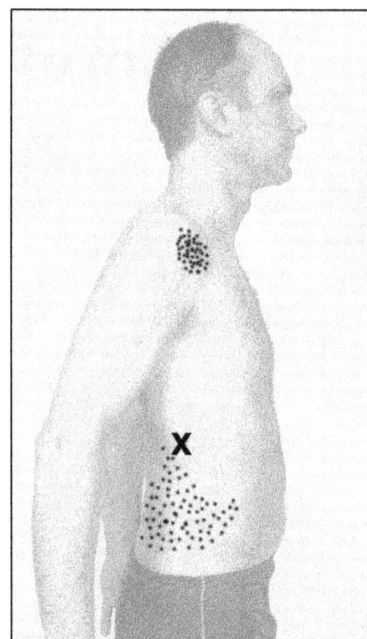

Causes and Perpetuation of Trigger Points
- carrying boxes or other heavy objects in front of you
- weight lifting or pulling weights down overhead
- hanging from a swing or rope
- weeding a garden
- a tight bra strap around your chest
- throwing heavy bags of laundry or other objects repeatedly
- aggressively swimming the butterfly stroke
- throwing a baseball
- working with a heavy chainsaw at shoulder level

This is a list of perpetuating factors specific only to trigger points in <u>this</u> *muscle. For a full list of perpetuating factors that can cause and perpetuate trigger points anywhere in the body and which also apply to this muscle, please see "Appendix A" (found at the end of this book), since some may need to be addressed for lasting pain relief.*

Helpful Hints
- Avoid reaching up and above to hold or retrieve objects. Use a foot stool or stepladder if necessary.
- At night, avoid drawing your arm tightly into your body. Instead, try to keep your elbow out away from your body. You may try putting a pillow next to your trunk to help with this.
- Wear bras that fit properly. If you see elastic marks on your skin after you take your bra off, the straps are too tight. Jogging bras work great for medium or small-breasted women. Have the salesperson help you find a bra that fits properly -- many of them really know their products.

- If you must pull down on something, keep your upper arm at your side.
- Referred pain from the *latissimus dorsi* and other muscles can be mis-diagnosed as "thoracic outlet syndrome." See *scalenes* (chapter 7) for a discussion of that syndrome and the other muscles that may be involved.

Self-Help Techniques

Check the *serratus posterior superior* (chapter 10), since pain referral from that muscle can cause trigger points in the *latissimus dorsi*.

Applying Pressure

Latissimus Dorsi Pressure: With the arm of the affected side resting on the back of a couch, use the opposite hand to reach under the armpit and pinch an area about one inch below the armpit. Be sure to pinch as close to the rib cage as possible, rather than just pinching a fold of skin. Pressing with the fingers may be more effective for some people and will be effective for reaching the lower trigger points too.

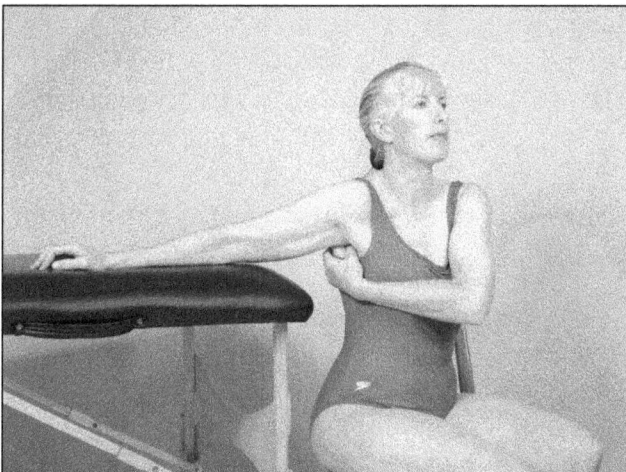

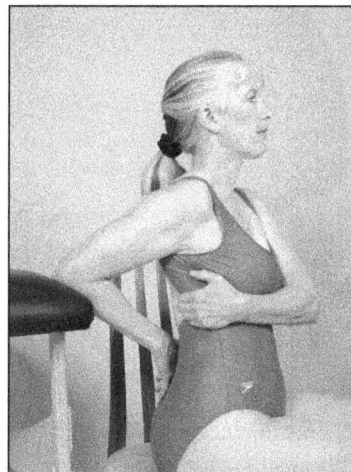

You may also try lying on a tennis or racquet ball if the muscle is not too tender. Lie on the bed, with your arm out straight above your head—the tender spot will likely be just below the armpit.

Stretches

Latissimus Dorsi Stretch: Wrap the hand of the affected side behind your head and, if possible, touch your fingers to your opposite ear. Reach even further forward if you are not forcing the stretch. Ideally you will eventually be able to reach all the way to the corner of your mouth.

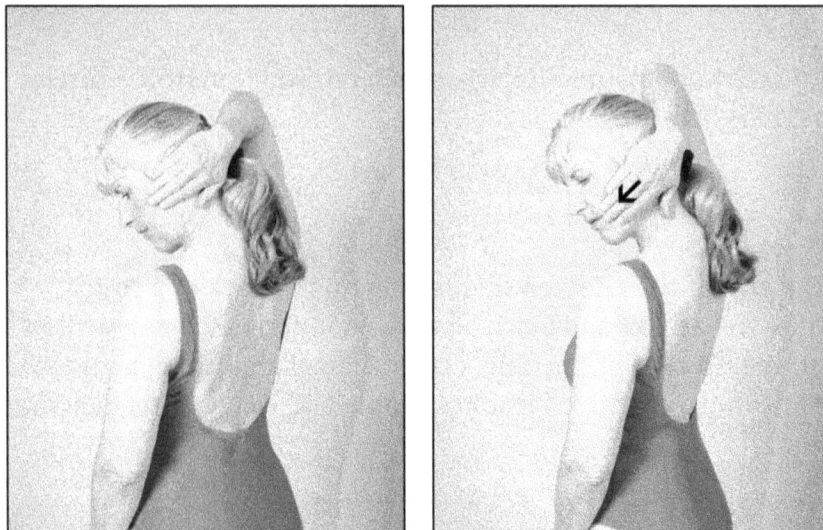

Pectoralis Stretch: Stretching the *pectoralis* muscles will help treat the *latissimus dorsi* muscle; see chapter 8.

Follow both stretches with a hot pack applied for 15 to 20 minutes. Lay the hot pack on you, rather than lying on the hot pack, which can cut off needed circulation and cause burns.

Also See:
* Triceps (satellite trigger points, chapter 18)
* Paraspinal (iliocostalis thoracis, satellite trigger points, chapter 4)
* Serratus posterior superior (chapter 10)
* Trapezius (lower portion, satellite trigger points, chapter 3)
* Subscapularis (chapter 14)

You may need to check the *teres major* (chapter 15) and *triceps* (chapter 18), since these muscles will often concurrently develop trigger points with the *latissimus dorsi*.

You may also need to work on the *serratus anterior, serratus posterior inferior, hand and finger flexors* (satellite trigger points) and abdominal muscles (*rectus abdominis*, upper portion) muscles to obtain complete relief, since trigger points in those muscles can either cause similar pain referral patterns or may affect or be affected by *latissimus dorsi* trigger points in some way.

Since trigger points in these muscles (with the exception of the *triceps*) don't directly cause shoulder pain, they are not addressed in this book. If you can't relieve your pain with the self-help techniques in this book after six to eight weeks, you may wish to consider whether you need to treat trigger points in these additional muscles, or if you still have perpetuating factors to resolve. Go to the end of this book for other books by the author that provide self-treatment techniques of muscles not covered in this book.

> **Differential Diagnosis:** If you are unable to relieve your symptoms with trigger point self-help techniques, you may need to see a health care provider to rule out entrapment of the suprascapular nerve at the spine of the scapula, a C_7 nerve root irritation, or an ulnar neuropathy, all diagnosed through electrodiagnostic examinations. Bicipital tendonitis may be caused by trigger points in the biceps muscle. You may need to see a chiropractor or osteopathic physician to be evaluated for innominate dysfunction or misalignment of any of the vertebrae between and including T_7 to L_4. The head of the humerus (upper arm bone) may need to be checked for its position in the shoulder joint.

Chapter 14: Subscapularis

The subscapularis is located on the anterior (front) surface of the shoulder blade, between the shoulder blade and the rib cage, making it difficult to access with finger pressure.

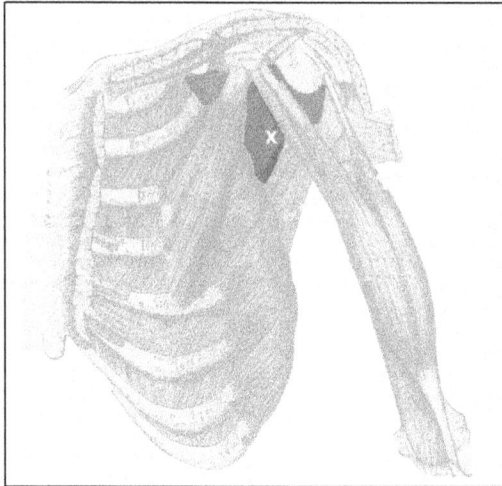

Front view of shoulder blade <u>through</u> front of trunk

This is one of four muscles that form the "rotator cuff," along with the *supraspinatus* (chapter 11), *infraspinatus* (chapter 12), and *teres minor* (chapter 16). For more information on rotator cuff injuries and frozen shoulder, see chapter 2. Pain is more often due to trigger points, and may also be present even if a tear is confirmed, especially if tightness in the muscle from trigger points contributed to the overload that lead to the tear.

Common Symptoms

- severe referred pain primarily over the back of the *deltoid* area, with possibly some referral over the shoulder blade, down the *triceps* area, and possibly a strap-like area of referred pain and tenderness around the wrist, worse on the back side
- restricted range of motion, often severely limited as the condition progresses
- an inability to reach backward with the arm at shoulder level, as when throwing a ball

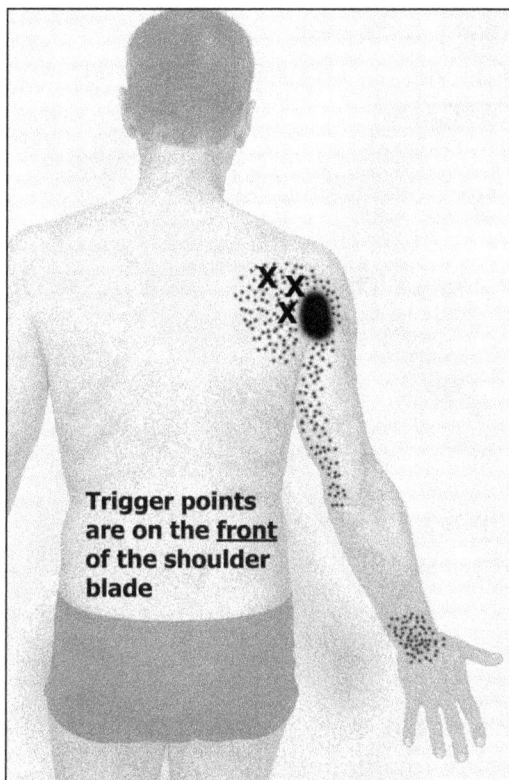

Rear referral pattern   *Front referral pattern*

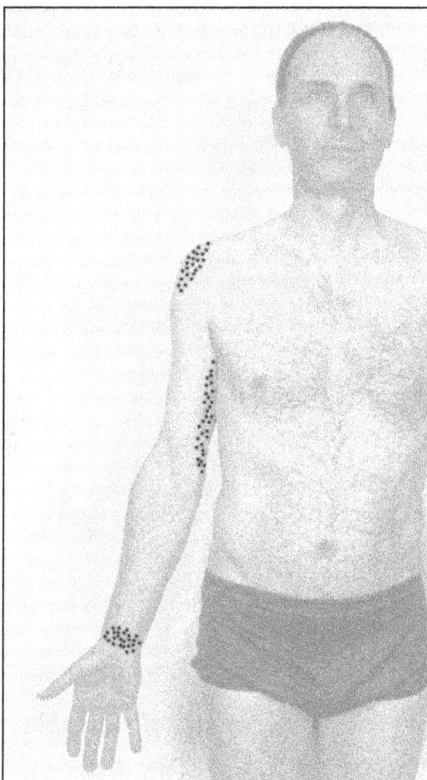

Causes and Perpetuation of Trigger Points

- overuse of muscles that aren't accustomed to repetitive motions, such as the crawl stroke or pitching a ball
- repeated forceful overhead lifting, as when swinging a child up and down
- slumped posture
- sudden trauma, such as reaching back to stop yourself from falling, catching an object from falling, dislocating your shoulder, breaking the upper arm, or by tearing the shoulder joint capsule
- long-term immobilization, such as in a cast and shoulder splint

This is a list of perpetuating factors specific only to trigger points in this muscle. For a full list of perpetuating factors that can cause and perpetuate trigger points anywhere in the body and which also apply to this muscle, please see "Appendix A" (found at the end of this book), since some may need to be addressed for lasting pain relief.

Helpful Hints

- When you sleep on the affected side or your back, use a pillow between your trunk and upper arm to keep your arm out at a 90-degree angle. When the affected side is toward the ceiling, drape your arm over a pillow.
- When sitting, move your arm frequently, resting it on the back of the couch or car seat, or an armrest. When standing, hook your thumb in your belt.

- Referred pain from the subscapularis and other muscles can be mis-diagnosed as "thoracic outlet syndrome." See the *scalene* muscle (chapter 7) for a discussion of that syndrome and the other muscles that may be involved.

Self-Help Techniques

Related trigger points may also be found in the *teres major* (chapter 15), *latissimus dorsi* (chapter 13), *pectoralis major* (chapter 8), *infraspinatus* (chapter 12), and *teres minor* (chapter 16), so be sure to also check those muscles.

Applying Pressure

Treating this muscle will require the assistance of a therapist of some kind, as the *subscapularis* is difficult to access on your own for applying pressure.

Stretches

Pectoralis Stretch: Stretching the *pectoralis* muscles will help treat the *subscapularis* muscle. After application of heat over the shoulder blade and pectoralis major areas, do the stretch in chapter 8.

You may also stretch this muscle by resting your arm across the back of a car seat or couch, by reaching your arm up and behind your head, or by reaching toward the ceiling.

Exercises

Subscapularis Exercise: Lean over with your arm hanging down and swing your arm in a wide circle in a clockwise direction for the left arm and a counter clockwise direction for the right arm. Be sure to keep your head totally relaxed.

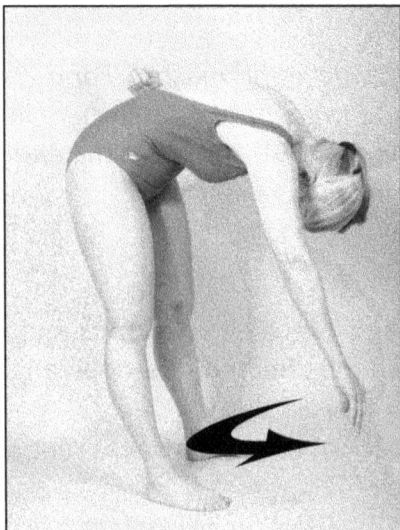

Also See:

* Pectoralis major (chapter 8)
* Teres major (chapter 15)
* Latissimus dorsi (chapter 13)
* Triceps (chapter 18, satellite trigger points)
* Deltoid (chapter 17, satellite trigger points)
* Supraspinatus (chapter 11)
* Infraspinatus (chapter 12)
* Teres minor (chapter 16)

The other muscles that typically get involved with the subscapularis in a frozen shoulder are the *pectoralis major* (chapter 8), *latissimus dorsi* (chapter 13), and *teres major* (chapter 15), so be sure to check these if you have restricted range-of-motion.

Differential Diagnosis: Pain from *subscapularis* trigger points can either mimic or occur concurrently with rotator cuff tears, adhesive capsulitis, a C_7 nerve root irritation, a true thoracic outlet syndrome, or a nerve impingement, so you may need to see a health care provider and undergo an MRI or other diagnostic tests to check for those conditions. In true adhesive capsulitis, an arthrogram contrast medium shows that the normally rounded outline of the capsule is replaced by a squat, square contracted patch, along with restrictions of the joint volume, serration of the bursal attachments, failure to fill the biceps tendon sheath, and partial obliteration of subscapular and axillary recesses. Adhesive capsulitis exhibits less pain and more rigidity than that caused by trigger points, and often requires short-term oral steroids. A rotator cuff tear causes severe pain and usually exhibits a limited arc of motion.

Chapter 15: Teres Major

The *teres major* forms the back "wall" of the armpit.

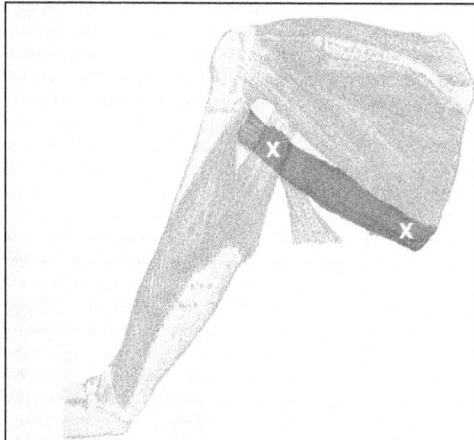
Back view of left shoulder blade

Common Symptoms

- primarily referred pain to the outside and back of the shoulder and over the back of the upper arm, and sometimes over the back of the forearm
- usually pain is felt when using the arm out in front, or when reaching forward and up
- a slight restriction in range of motion when reaching overhead, but for most people not likely a noticeable amount
- if the posterior *deltoid*, *teres minor*, and *subscapularis* also develop trigger points, range of motion can be greatly restricted and the shoulder area can become very painful, resulting in "frozen shoulder" (see chapter 2 for a discussion of "frozen shoulder")

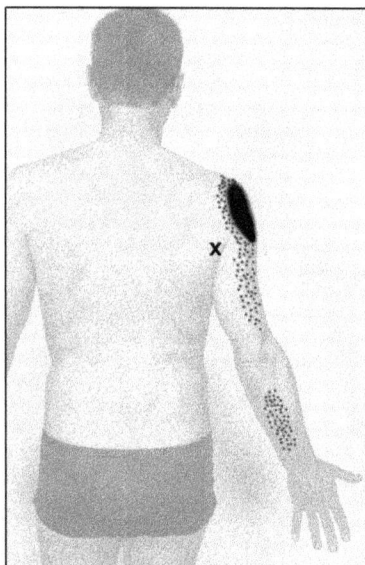
Back referral pattern

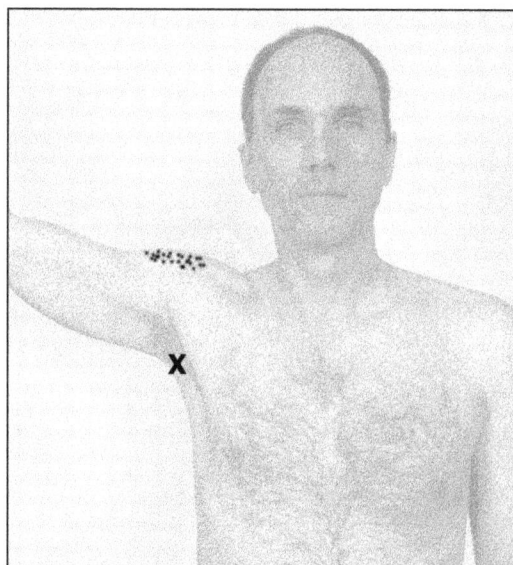
Front referral pattern

Causes and Perpetuation of Trigger Points

- any activity that requires sustained resistance, such as driving a car that is hard to steer
- lifting weights overhead
- massage therapists who use their elbows
- dancing with a partner who forces his partners' arms into position

This is a list of perpetuating factors specific only to trigger points in <u>this</u> muscle. For a full list of perpetuating factors that can cause and perpetuate trigger points anywhere in the body and which also apply to this muscle, please see "Appendix A" (found at the end of this book), since some may need to be addressed for lasting pain relief.

Helpful Hints

- Avoid strenuous activities that aggravate trigger points in the *teres major* (such as lifting weights overhead) until self-help techniques have lessened the pain substantially.
- Be sure your car is easy to steer, or that any activity you perform on a regular basis is modified until it no longer causes trigger point activation.
- Drape the affected arm over a pillow at night.
- Referred pain from the *teres major* and other muscles can be mis-diagnosed as "thoracic outlet syndrome." See the *scalene* muscle (chapter 7) for a discussion of that syndrome and the other muscles that may be involved.

Self-Help Techniques

Trigger points will also usually be found in the *latissimus dorsi* (chapter 13) and *triceps* (chapter 18) muscles. If the posterior *deltoid* (chapter 17), *teres minor* (chapter 16), and *subscapularis* (chapter 14) muscles also become involved and result in a painful frozen shoulder, then you will need to check and work on those muscles too.

Relieving *teres major* trigger points may release tightness in the *rhomboid* muscle (chapter 5), which may develop trigger points as a result of a tight *teres major* pulling on the mid back area.

Applying Pressure

Teres Major Pressure: Lie on your side and extend your arm so that it is sticking straight up above your head. Remember, the *teres major* forms the back wall of the armpit, so be sure you are working on that area.

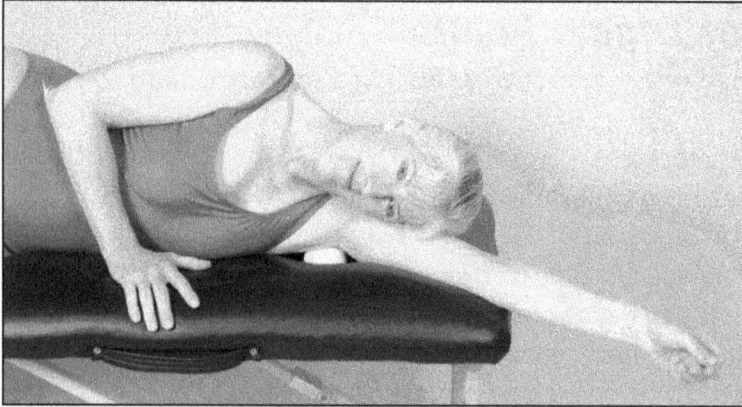

You may also rest the arm on the back of a couch or adjacent chair and "pinch" the muscle in between your thumb and fingers.

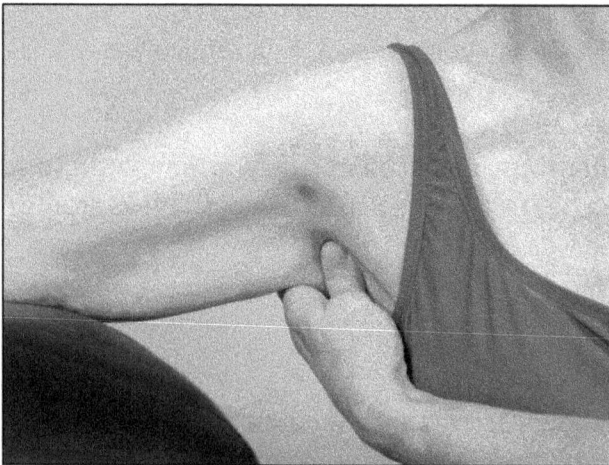

Stretches

Triceps Stretch: The stretch for the *triceps* also benefits the *teres major* (see chapter 18).

Also See:
* Latissimus dorsi (chapter 13)
* Triceps (chapter 18)
* Deltoid (chapter 17, posterior portion)
* Teres minor (chapter 16)
* Subscapularis (chapter 14)

Differential Diagnosis: If you are unable to relieve your symptoms with trigger point self-help techniques, you may need to see a health care provider to be evaluated for subacromial or subdeltoid bursitis, supraspinatus tendonitis, C_6 or C_7 nerve root irritation, and *true* thoracic outlet syndrome, any of which can cause similar pain patterns.

Chapter 16: Teres Minor

The *teres minor* is one of the four muscles forming the "rotator cuff," along with the *infraspinatus* (chapter 12), *supraspinatus* (chapter 11), and *subscapularis* (chapter 14), and usually only harbors trigger points if the *infraspinatus* is also involved.

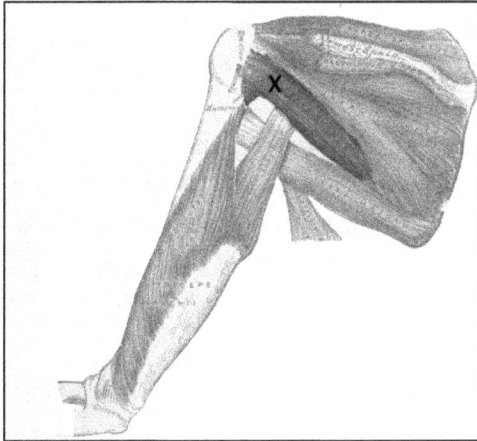

Back view of left shoulder blade

See chapter 2 for more information on "rotator cuff injuries." Pain is more often due to trigger points, and may also be present even if a tear is confirmed, especially if tightness in the muscle from trigger points contributed to the overload that lead to the tear.

Common Symptoms

- deep localized pain in the posterior *deltoid* (chapter 17), which is likely only noticeable after *infraspinatus* (chapter 12) trigger points have been inactivated.
- possibly numbness and tingling of the ring and little fingers, which is aggravated by reaching above shoulder height or behind your body

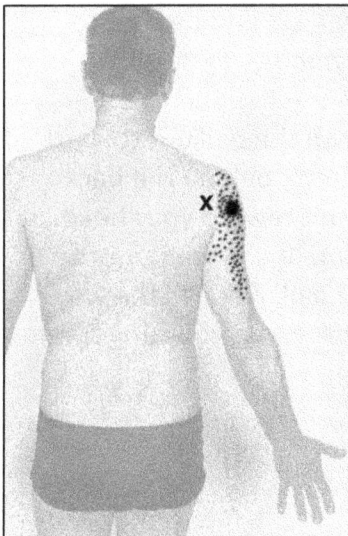

Causes and Perpetuation of Trigger Points

- a sudden overload of the muscle by arresting yourself from a fall or trying to hold onto something heavy
- anything that requires you to hold your arms out in front of or above you for extended periods of time with the arms not well supported, such as computer use (especially your "mouse arm"), kayaking, driving, or tennis
- reaching behind you
- holding onto something such as the steering wheel during an auto accident
- trigger points are usually found in conjunction with *infraspinatus* trigger points

This is a list of perpetuating factors specific only to trigger points in this *muscle. For a full list of perpetuating factors that can cause and perpetuate trigger points anywhere in the body and which also apply to this muscle, please see "Appendix A" (found at the end of this book), since some may need to be addressed for lasting pain relief.*

Helpful Hints

- Modify or replace your mis-fitting furniture. Your knees should fit under your desk, and the chair needs to be close enough that you can lean against your backrest. Your elbows should rest on either your work surface or armrests at the same height. Your elbows and forearms should rest evenly on the armrests. Your computer screen should be directly in front of you, and the copy attached to the side of the screen, so that you may look directly forward as much as possible.
- Sleep with your arm out at a 90-degree angle, and put a pillow between your upper arm and trunk if necessary. Apply a hot pack to the back wall of your armpit before bedtime.

Self-Help Techniques

Applying Pressure

Infraspinatus Pressure: Read the *infraspinatus* muscle chapter (chapter 12) and be sure to perform the self-help on that muscle first before working on the *teres minor*.

Teres Minor Pressure: After working on the *infraspinatus*, continue with the ball out toward the upper arm. The muscle is in the dip between the trunk and upper arm, behind the back wall of the armpit. Lie on your side with your arm extended up a little bit toward your head. If you want less pressure, put your head on a pillow *behind* the upper arm. If you want more pressure, rest your head *on* your upper arm. Using a tennis or racquet ball, work all the way from the outer edge of the shoulder blade to about a quarter of the way down your upper arm.

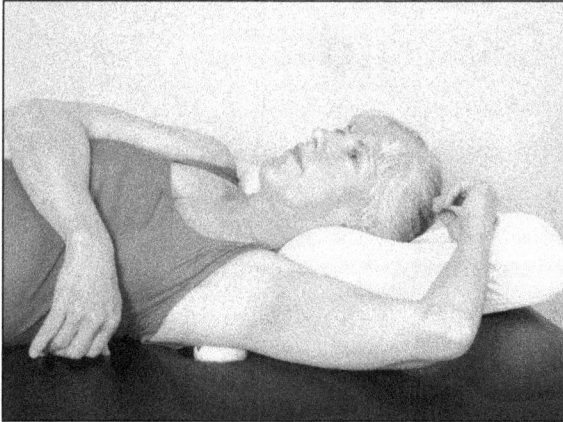

Stretches

Teres Minor Stretch: Stretch by grasping the affected arm above the elbow and bring your arm up and across your face.

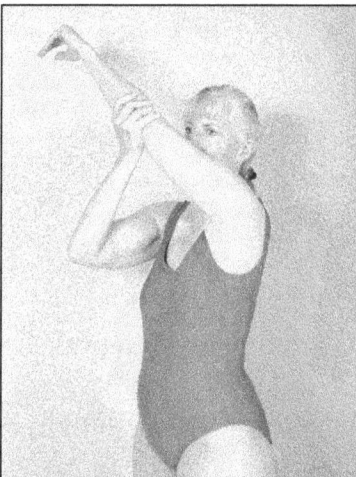

Also See:
* Infraspinatus (chapter 12)

Differential Diagnosis: If you are unable to relieve your symptoms with trigger point self-help techniques, you may need to see a health care provider for further diagnostic testing. Symptoms of quadrilateral space syndrome include shoulder pain and selective atrophy of the teres minor muscle due to compression of the axillary nerve by fibrous bands as it passes through the quadrilateral space, and can be diagnosed by an MRI. Numbness and tingling of the ring and little fingers can be confused with ulnar neuropathy or C_8 nerve root irritation, and can be diagnosed by an electrodiagnostic evaluation. Subdeltoid bursitis can cause symptoms similar to pain referred from teres minor trigger points. If there has been an impactful injury, an acromioclavicular separation may need to be ruled out. A rotator cuff tear causes severe pain and usually exhibits a limited arc of motion, and must be confirmed by an MRI, arthrogram, or ultrasound.

Chapter 17: Deltoid

The *deltoid* muscle is located at the top end of the upper arm, attaching at the top around the front, back, and side of the area around the shoulder socket, and at the bottom coming to a point in about the middle of the outside upper arm. Trigger points in the *deltoid* are common, and are frequently due to satellite trigger points from other muscles.

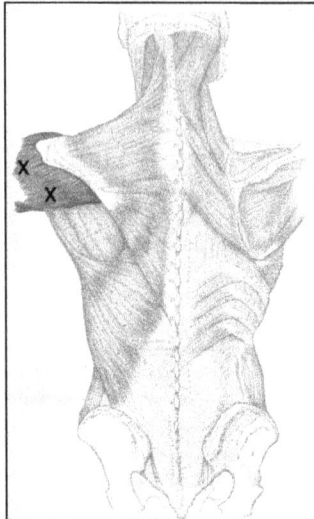

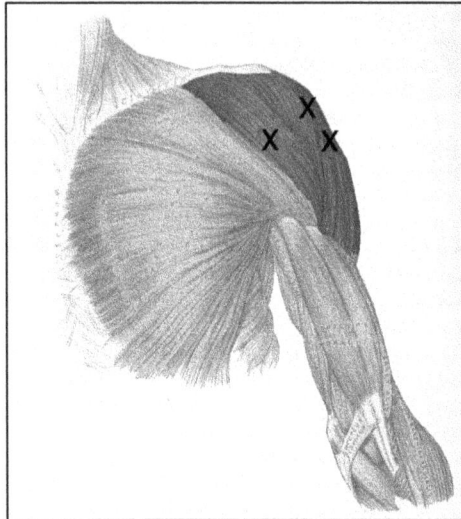

Front view of left shoulder

Common Symptoms

- pain is usually localized in the *deltoid* muscle area, at its worst with the arm in motion, with deep, less intense pain at rest
- restricted range of motion, most often raising it more than 90-degrees to the front or sides, but it can be less than 90-degrees in severe cases
- possibly loss of strength

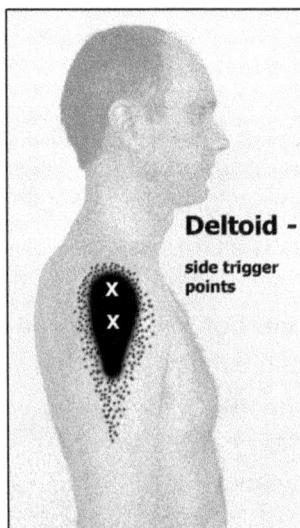

Deltoid -

side trigger points

Deltoid -
back trigger
point

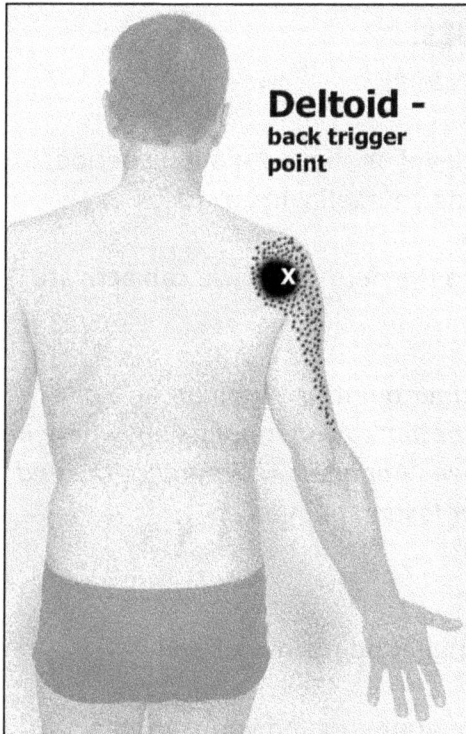

Back trigger point, back referral pattern

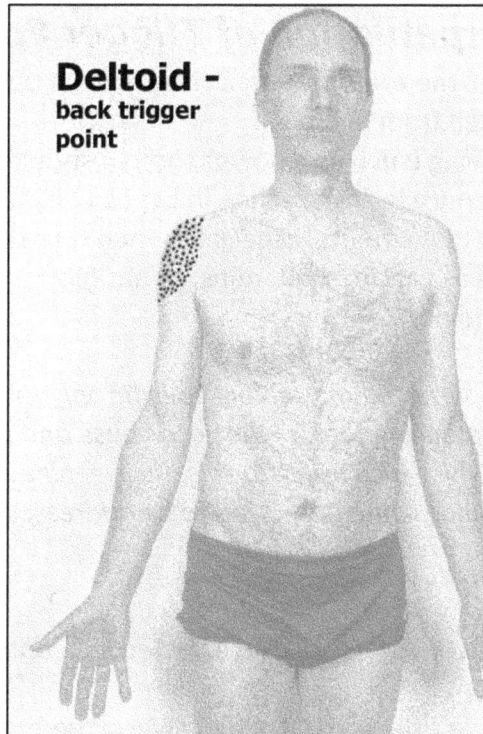

Deltoid -
back trigger
point

Back trigger point, front referral pattern

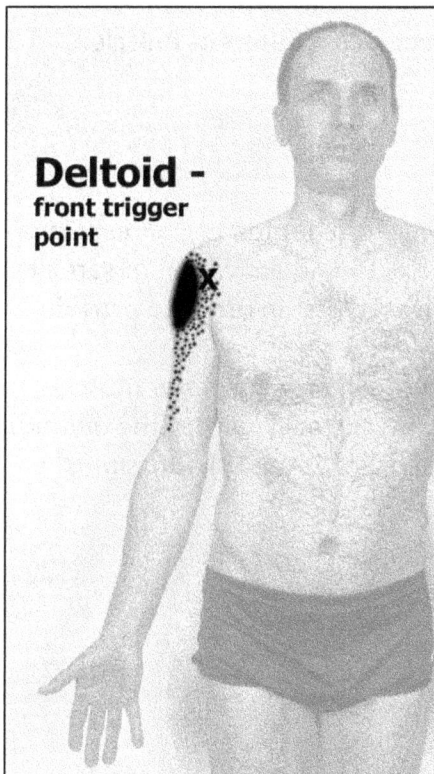

Deltoid -
front trigger
point

Front trigger point, front referral pattern

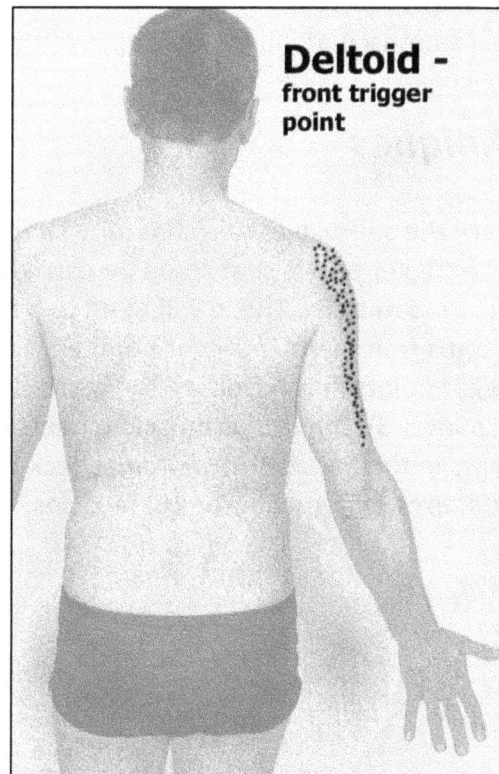

Deltoid -
front trigger
point

Front trigger point, back referral pattern

Causes and Perpetuation of Trigger Points

- a direct blow to the area, as with a rifle recoil or sports injury
- catching yourself from a fall
- holding something (such as a power tool) at shoulder level or above for a long period
- overuse of the muscle as in reeling in big fish or pushing yourself with ski poles
- vigorous, jerky movements, especially when repetitive
- injections such as vaccines, vitamins, or antibiotics into the *deltoid* muscle can activate latent trigger points

This is a list of perpetuating factors specific only to trigger points in this muscle. For a full list of perpetuating factors that can cause and perpetuate trigger points anywhere in the body and which also apply to this muscle, please see "Appendix A" (found at the end of this book), since some may need to be addressed for lasting pain relief.

Helpful Hints

- Avoid lifting heavy objects on the affected side until trigger points have been inactivated.
- If you are firing a rifle, place a pad between the butt of your gun and your shoulder.
- Be careful going down stairs, to prevent a near-fall. Hold onto the railing, and watch your feet placement carefully.
- If you receive intramuscular injections, see if you can inject into a different muscle.

Self-Help Techniques

Be sure to check the *supraspinatus* (chapter 11), *infraspinatus* (chapter 12), and *scalene* (chapter 7) muscles for trigger points that could be causing referral to and activation of satellite trigger points in the *deltoid* muscle. These will need to be inactivated first in order to provide lasting relief of symptoms from *deltoid* trigger points.

If you find trigger points in the front of the *deltoid*, check the *pectoralis major* muscle close to the armpit (chapter 8), the *biceps* muscle (chapter 19), and the back part of the *deltoid*. If you find trigger points in the back of the *deltoid*, check the *triceps* (chapter 18), *latissimus dorsi* (chapter 13), and *teres major* (chapter 15) muscles.

Applying Pressure

Deltoid Pressure: Use a tennis ball in a doorjamb. Place the ball in a lip of the doorjamb to help stabilize the ball, and keep holding the ball in your opposite hand so the ball doesn't slip away from you as you search for trigger points. Be sure to work the front, side, and back of the muscle, and from the top to bottom, to apply pressure to the entire *deltoid* muscle.

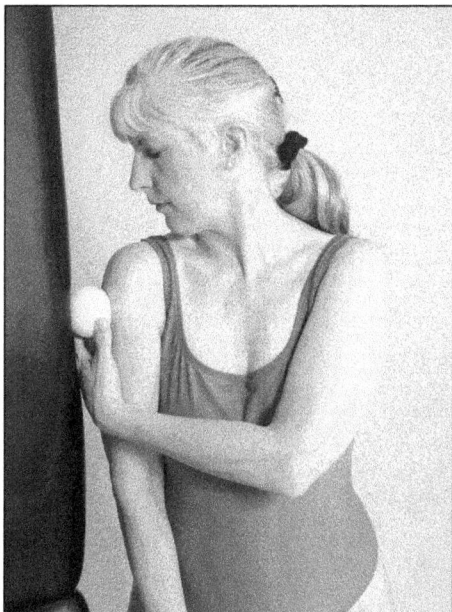

Stretches

Couch Stretch: Stretch the front part of the muscle by placing your arm over the back of a couch and rotating your shoulder forward.

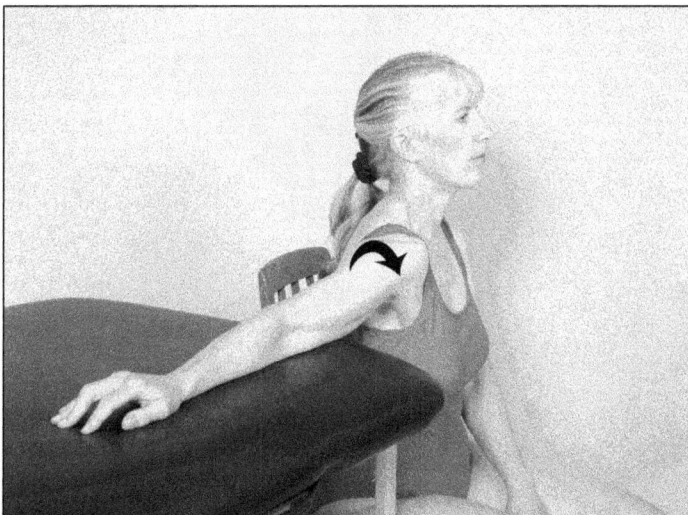

Against-Doorjamb Stretch: Stand in a doorway with your arm straightened at or slightly higher than 90°, with your palm on the doorjamb and your thumb pointing down. Put the foot of the same side as your arm about one step in front of you, and rotate your body gently away from your hand. As you rotate your shoulder forward and down, you'll feel the stretch move into the front portion of the *deltoid*, the *coracobrachialis*, and the *biceps* muscles.

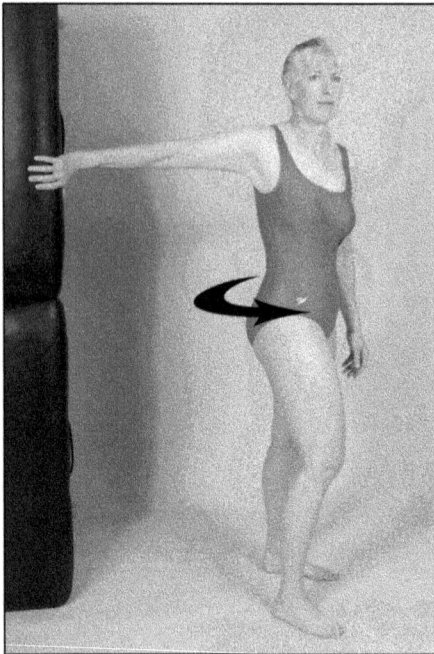

Posterior Deltoid Stretch: For the posterior portion of the *deltoid* muscle, pull your arm across your chest, using the opposite hand to grasp your arm near the elbow.

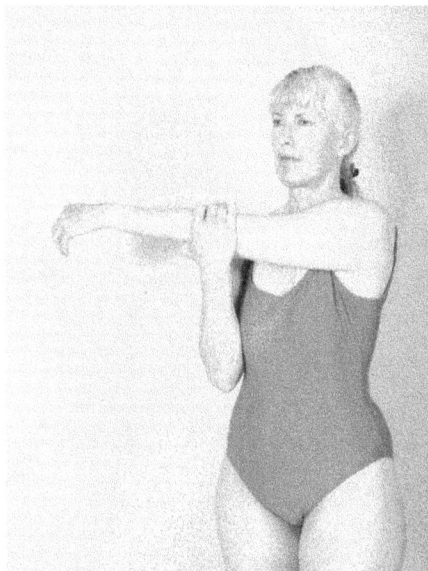

Pectoralis Stretch: Perform the middle and lower positions of the *pectoralis* stretch, which will also help treat the *deltoid* muscle (see chapter 8).

Also See:

* Pectoralis major (chapter 8)
* Biceps (chapter 19)
* Triceps (chapter 18)
* Latissimus dorsi (chapter 13)
* Teres major (chapter 15)
* Infraspinatus (chapter 12)
* Supraspinatus (chapter 11)
* Scalene (chapter 7)

Differential Diagnosis: Trigger points in the deltoid muscle are commonly misdiagnosed as rotator cuff tears, bicipital tendonitis, subdeltoid bursitis, glenohumeral joint arthritis, a nerve impingement, or a C_5 nerve root irritation. If you are unable to relieve your pain with the trigger point self-help, you may need to see a health care provider for an MRI, x-ray, or other diagnostic test to confirm or rule out the above diagnoses. Even if you do have one of these conditions, it is likely there are also trigger points involved.

If the shoulder joint is sprained, dislocated, separated, or out of alignment, there will be localized tenderness only over the joint rather than in the deltoid muscle, unless you also have trigger points that were present prior to the acute injury which also cause tenderness.

Chapter 18: Triceps • Anconeus

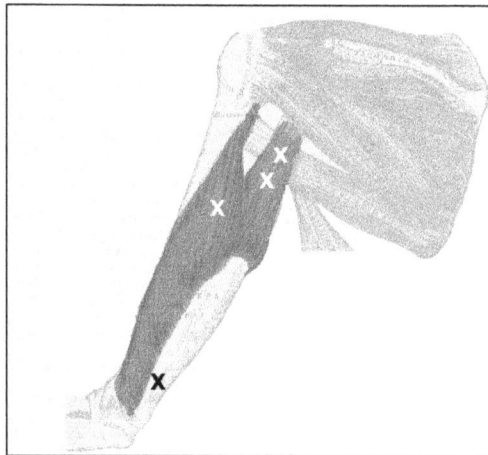

Triceps, back of left upper arm

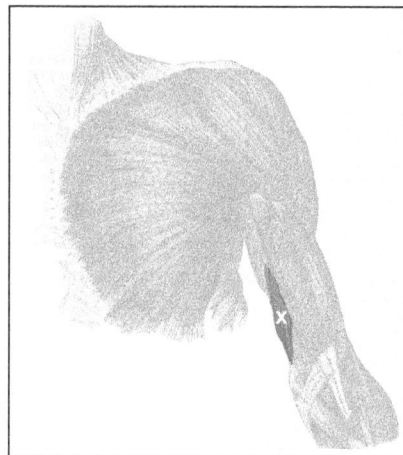

Triceps, front of left upper arm

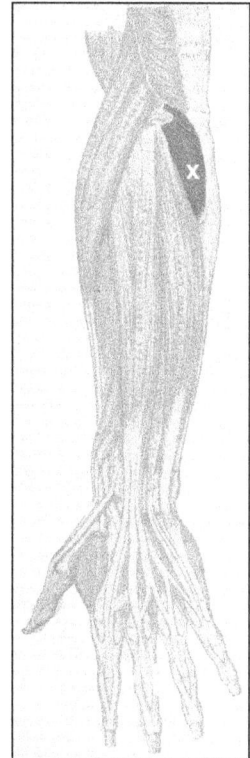

Anconeus, back view of lower left arm

Common Symptoms

- see the pictures for all the various pain referral patterns
- pain around the elbow is one of the most common referral patterns, and often causes and perpetuates trigger points in adjacent muscles
- pain from some trigger points may only be activated during certain sports that require full forceful extension at the elbow, such as tennis and golf
- possibly pain with pressing or tapping on one of the bony parts of the elbow
- if the *triceps* entraps the radial nerve, you may get tingling and numbness over the back of the lower forearm, wrist, and hand to the middle finger

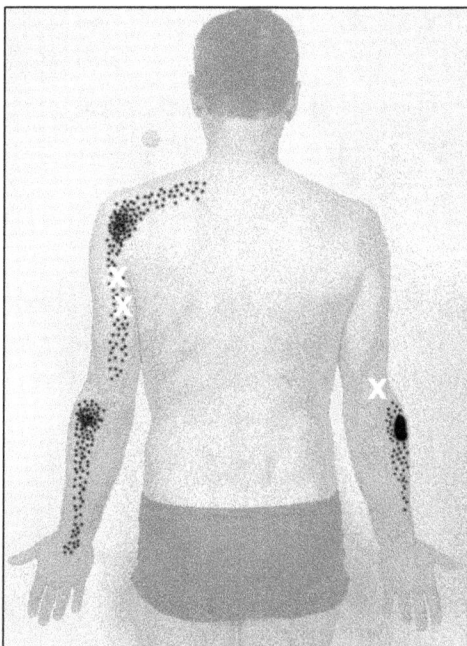

Triceps trigger points and referral patterns

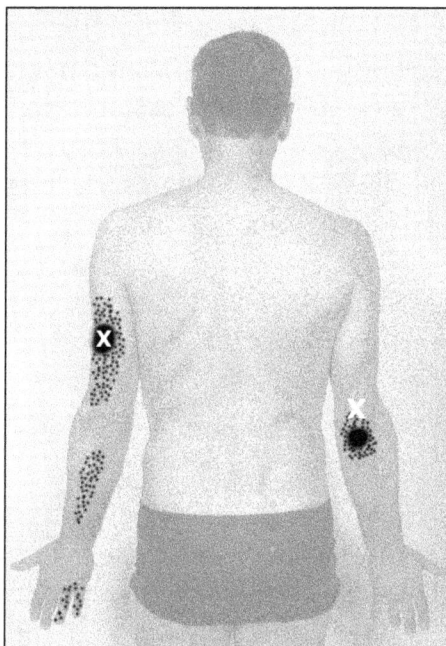

Triceps trigger points and referral patterns

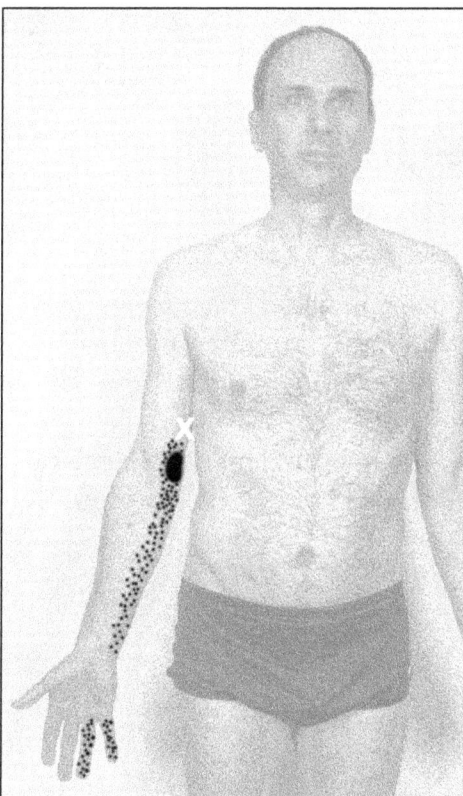

Triceps trigger points and referral patterns

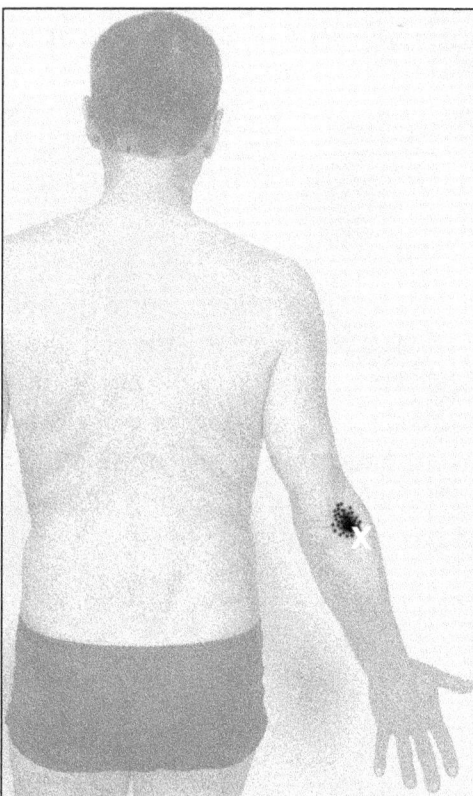

Anconeus trigger points and referral patterns

Causes and Perpetuation of Trigger Points

- sports strains (i.e., tennis, golf)
- excessive conditioning (i.e., push-ups, chin-ups)
- driving for long periods, especially excessive manual gear shifting

- hand-sewing without elbow support
- using a computer without proper arm supports
- a profession that requires a lot of pressure with the arms, such as massage therapy
- repetitively pressing bound books onto a copy machine
- using forearm crutches, or a cane that is too long
- anatomically short upper arms

This is a list of perpetuating factors specific only to trigger points in <u>these</u> muscles. For a full list of perpetuating factors that can cause and perpetuate trigger points anywhere in the body and which also apply to these muscles, please see "Appendix A" (found at the end of this book), since some may need to be addressed for lasting pain relief.

Helpful Hints

- Keep your upper arms by your side as much as possible when typing, writing, reading, and sewing, and use armrests of a proper height whenever possible (you shouldn't have to lean to the side -- the arms should be at the height of your elbow).
- Use a lighter tennis racquet or shorten the grip.
- Avoid chin-ups and push-ups.
- Start using forearm crutches gradually, if at all possible.

Self-Help Techniques

Applying Pressure

Triceps Pressure: Lie on your side with your arm extended above your head. If you want less pressure, put your head on a pillow *behind* the upper arm. If you want more pressure, rest your head *on* your upper arm. Using a tennis or racquet ball, rest your upper arm on the ball, working all the way from the back of your shoulder down to your elbow. Be sure to treat the front and back edges of the muscle too, by rotating the arm a little in both directions, since this muscle covers the entire back of the upper arm and trigger points can be found throughout the muscle. You may also pinch this muscle.

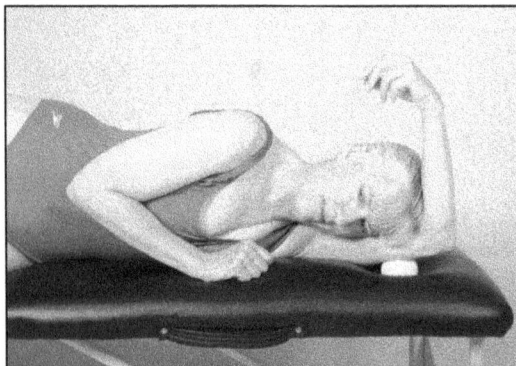

Stretches

Triceps Stretch: Standing sideways to the wall, place your elbow on the wall above your head, with your forearm bent and your hand behind your head. Lean slightly into the wall to get a gentle stretch.

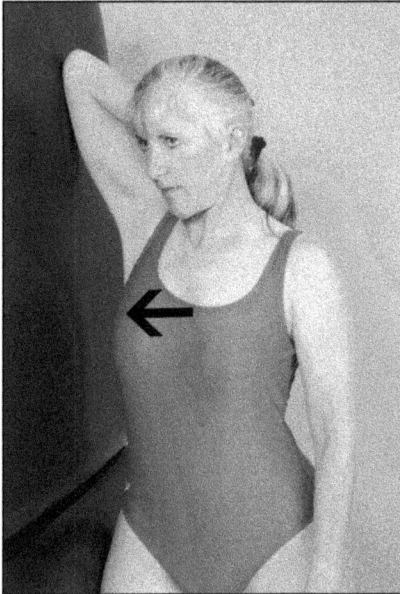

Also See:
* Latissimus dorsi (chapter 13)
* Serratus posterior superior (chapter 10)
* Teres major (chapter 15)
* Teres minor (chapter 16)
* Biceps (chapter 19)

You may also need to work on the *supinator, brachialis,* and hand extensors (*extensor carpi radialis longus and brachioradialis*) muscles to obtain complete relief.

Since trigger points in these muscles don't directly cause shoulder pain, they are not addressed in this book. If you can't relieve your pain with the self-help techniques in this book after six to eight weeks, you may wish to consider whether you need to treat trigger points in these additional muscles, or if you still have perpetuating factors to resolve. Go to the end of this book for other books by the author that provide self-treatment techniques of muscles not covered in this book.

Differential Diagnosis: Referred pain from triceps trigger points may be misdiagnosed as tennis elbow, tendonitis, lateral or medial epicondylitis, olecranon bursitis, thoracic outlet syndrome, arthritis, or a C$_7$ nerve root irritation, though these may occur concurrently. If trigger point self-help techniques don't relieve your pain, you may need to see a health care provider to rule out these conditions.

Chapter 19: Biceps

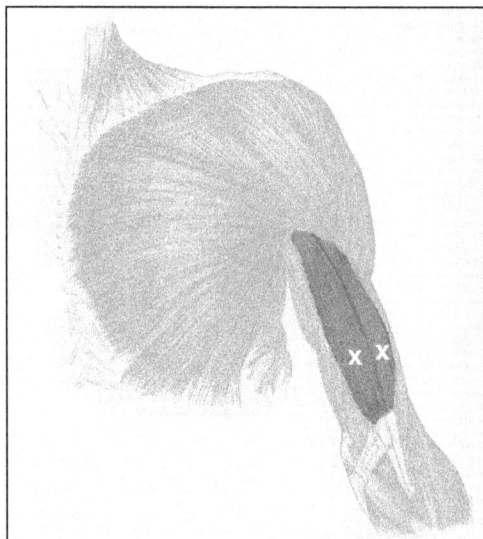

Front view of upper left arm

Common Symptoms

- trigger points are typically found in the mid-to-lower part of the muscle, and refer superficial achy pain over the front of the upper arm and front of the shoulder
- weakness and pain with raising the hand above the head with the elbow bent
- possibly an ache or soreness over the upper *trapezius* (top of the shoulder; see chapter 3) or the crease of the elbow

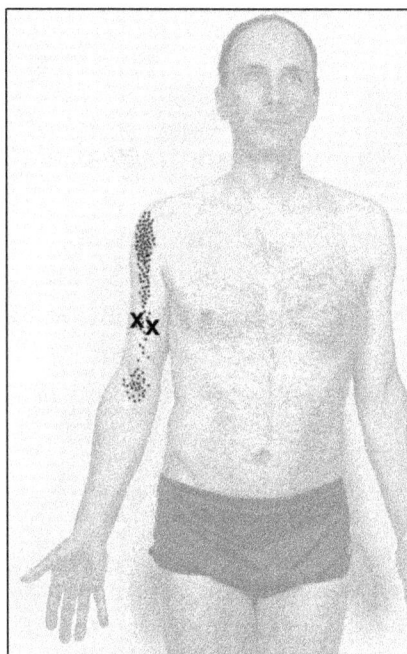

Front referral pattern

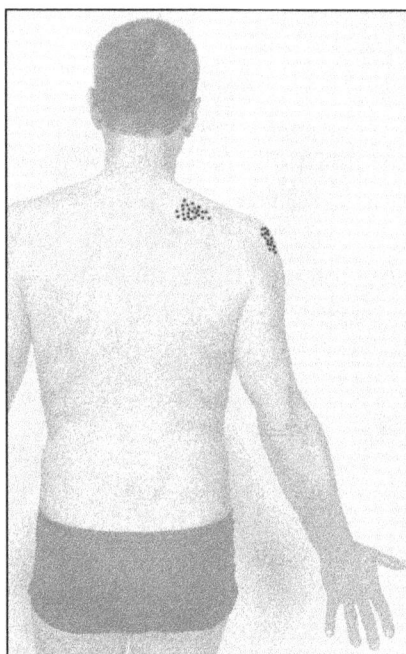

Back referral pattern

Causes and Perpetuation of Trigger Points

- throwing a ball or playing basketball or tennis
- writing, either with a pen or keyboard
- lifting heavy objects with your palms facing upward and/or with your arms extended forward, or shoveling snow
- playing the violin or guitar
- using a screwdriver for a long period
- trying to catch yourself from falling
- trigger points in the *infraspinatus* muscle (chapter 12) can cause satellite trigger points in the *biceps*

This is a list of perpetuating factors specific only to trigger points in <u>this</u> muscle. For a full list of perpetuating factors that can cause and perpetuate trigger points anywhere in the body and which also apply to this muscle, please see "Appendix A" (found at the end of this book), since some may need to be addressed for lasting pain relief.

Helpful Hints

- At night, don't draw your arm tightly into your body. Instead, try to keep your elbow out from your body. You may try putting a pillow in the crook of your elbow to help with this.
- Carry items either with your palms down, or in a daypack.

Self-Help Techniques

Applying Pressure

Biceps Pressure: With the opposite hand, either pinch the *biceps* between the thumb and next two fingers or just use your thumb to apply pressure.

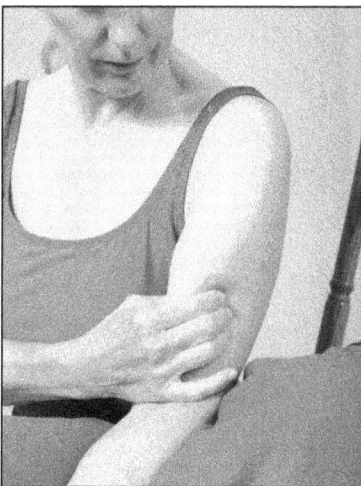

Stretches

Against-Doorjamb Stretch: The against-doorjamb stretch (chapter 17) will help treat the *biceps* muscle.

Also See:

*   Infraspinatus (chapter 12)
*   Triceps (chapter 18)
*   Deltoid (chapter 17, front portion)
*   Supraspinatus (chapter 11)
*   Trapezius (chapter 3, upper portion)
*   Coracobrachialis (chapter 20)

       Trigger points in the *triceps* (chapter 18), *deltoid* (front portion, chapter 17), *supraspinatus* (chapter 11), *trapezius* (upper portion, chapter 3), and *coracobrachialis* (chapter 20) muscles usually develop concurrently or within a few weeks' time of *biceps* trigger points, so you should also check those muscles.

       Trigger points in the *brachialis* and *supinator* muscles also usually develop concurrently or within a few weeks' time of *biceps* trigger points, but since trigger points in these muscles don't directly cause shoulder pain, they are not addressed in this book. If you can't relieve your pain with the self-help techniques in this book after six to eight weeks, you may wish to consider whether you need to treat trigger points in these additional muscles, or if you still have perpetuating factors to resolve. Go to the end of this book for other books by the author that provide self-treatment techniques of muscles not covered in this book.

Differential Diagnosis: If you are unable to relieve your symptoms with trigger point self-help techniques, you may need to see a health care provider for an MRI, x-ray, or other test to rule out or confirm a diagnosis of bicipital tendonitis, subdeltoid bursitis, C_5 nerve root irritation, bicipital bursitis, and glenohumeral arthritis.

Chapter 20: Coracobrachialis

The *coracobrachialis* muscle is on the front of the shoulder, in the crease between the trunk and the upper arm. Not everyone has this muscle. This is a good one to check if you have already searched for and inactivated trigger points in the *deltoid, pectoralis major, latissimus dorsi, teres major, supraspinatus, triceps,* and *biceps,* and have not gotten total relief.

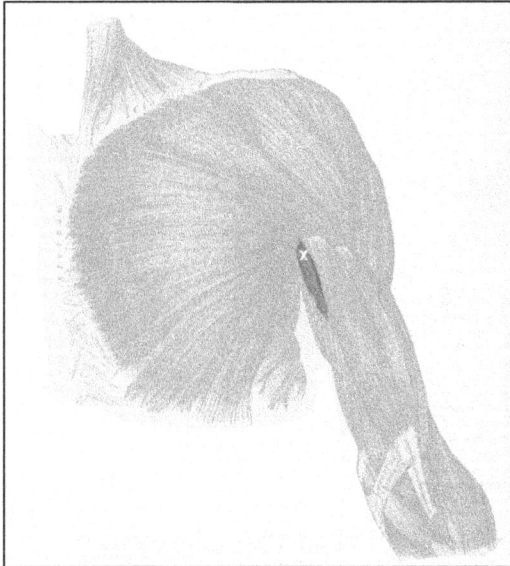

Front view of left upper arm

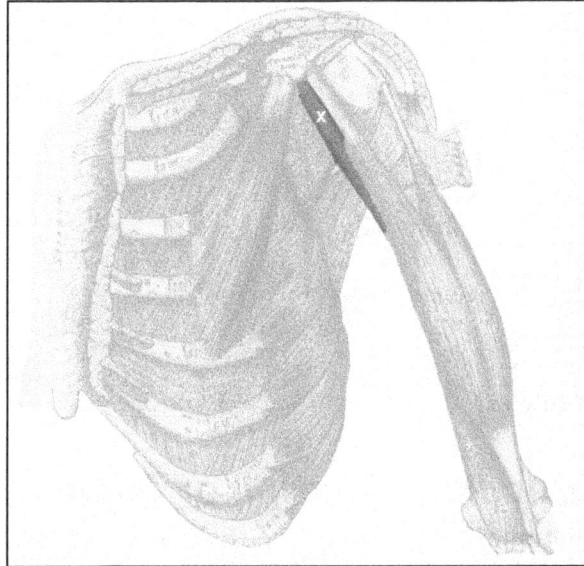

Left upper arm with the pectoralis major removed in order to get a better view of the coracobrachialis

Common Symptoms

- pain referred to the anterior *deltoid* (chapter 17), over the *triceps* (chapter 18) on the back of the upper arm, down the back of the lower arm, and sometimes into the back of the hand and middle finger
- if *only* the *coracobrachialis* is involved, pain is felt when reaching forward and up above past the ear without the elbow bent, and range-of-motion is restricted
- when placing the affected arm in the small of your back, it is difficult to get your hand past your spine without pain, whereas normally you should be able to touch the opposite arm with your fingers
- an entrapment of the musculocutaneous nerve as it passes through the *coracobrachialis* muscle may cause atrophy of the *biceps* muscle and reduced sensation on the back of the lower arm

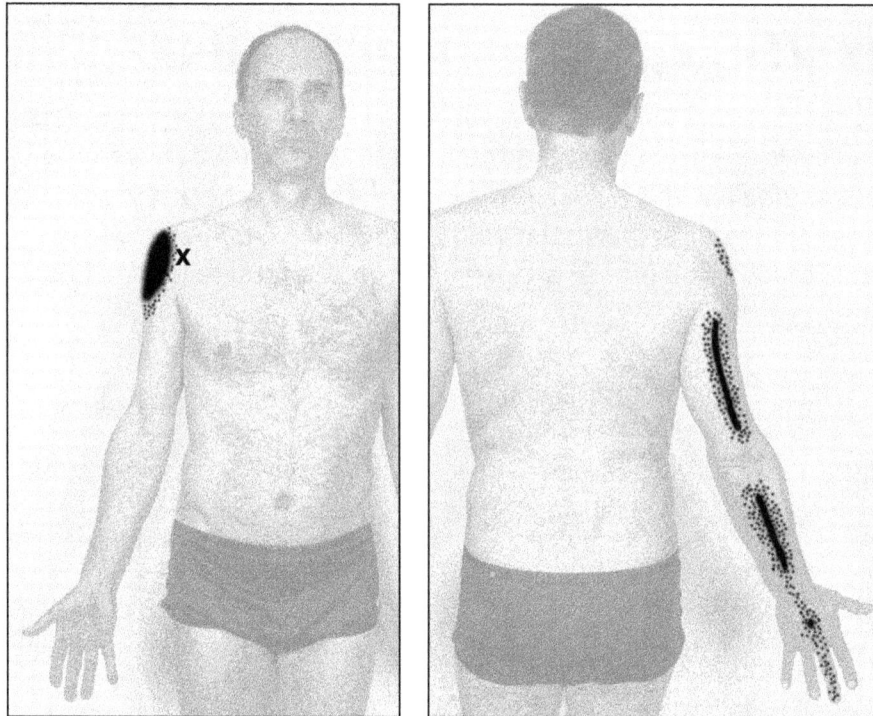

Front referral pattern   **Back referral pattern**

Causes and Perpetuation of Trigger Points

- activation of trigger points in the *coracobrachialis* occur only as a satellite area to the *deltoid, pectoralis major, latissimus dorsi, teres major, supraspinatus, triceps,* and *biceps* muscles, so these need to be relieved first for lasting relief in the coracobrachialis muscle (see below for chapter numbers).

   This is a list of perpetuating factors specific only to trigger points in <u>this</u> muscle. For a full list of perpetuating factors that can cause and perpetuate trigger points anywhere in the body and which also apply to this muscle, please see "Appendix A" (found at the end of this book), since some may need to be addressed for lasting pain relief.

Helpful Hints

- When lifting, hold objects close to your body, with your palms face-up as much as possible.

Self-Help Techniques

   Check the *deltoid* (chapter 17), *triceps* (chapter 18), *pectoralis major* (chapter 8), *latissimus dorsi* (chapter 13), *supraspinatus* (chapter 11), *teres major* (chapter 15), and *biceps* (chapter 19) muscles first, and relieve any trigger points as needed.

Applying Pressure

Coracobrachialis Pressure: Using the hand of the unaffected side, wrap your fingers around the deltoid. With your thumb knuckle bent, dig the end of your thumb into the front of the shoulder on the outside of the crease, pressing toward the bone in the upper arm. Some of my patients have found they prefer to use something like a pressure gadget of some kind; these are often sold in massage stores or catalogs, or see www.pressurepositive.com.

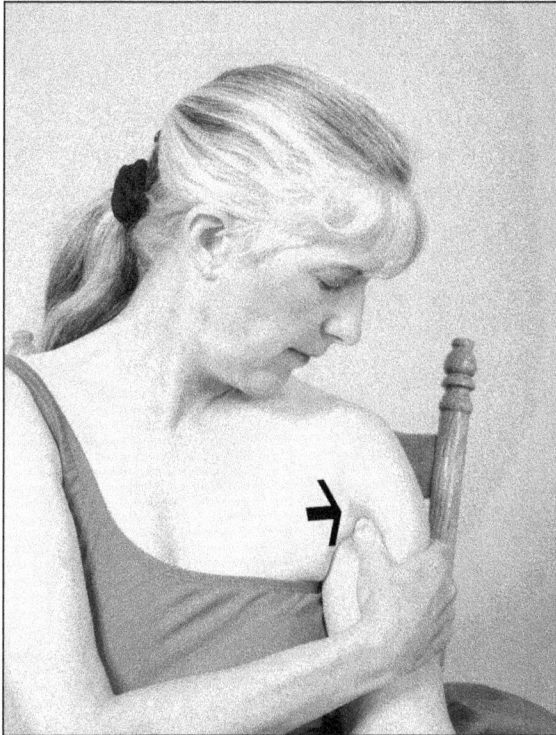

Stretches

Warm the area on the front of your shoulder/crease with moist heat before performing these stretches.

Pectoralis Stretch: Use the *pectoralis* stretch, lower hand position (see chapter 8).

Couch Stretch: See chapter 17 for this stretch.

Against-Doorjamb Stretch: See chapter 17 for this stretch. As you rotate your shoulder forward and down, you'll feel the stretch move into the front portion of the *deltoid* and the *coracobrachialis*.

Also See:

* Supraspinatus (chapter 11)
* Deltoid (chapter 17)
* Triceps (chapter 18)
* Biceps   (chapter 19)
* Pectoralis major (chapter 8)
* Teres major (chapter 15)
* Latissimus dorsi (chapter 13)

Differential Diagnosis: Symptoms from trigger points in the coracobrachialis muscle can be similar to C_7 nerve root irritation, carpal tunnel syndrome, subacromial bursitis, supraspinatus tendonitis, and acromioclavicular joint dysfunction. If you are unable to relieve your symptoms with trigger point self-help, you may need to see a health care provider for an MRI, x-ray, or other diagnostic test to confirm or rule out one of those diagnoses.

APPENDIX A

What Causes and Keeps Trigger Points Going: Perpetuating Factors

"If we treat myofascial pain syndromes without . . . correcting the multiple perpetuating factors, the patient is doomed to endless cycles of treatment and relapse. [Perpetuating factors are] the most neglected part of the management of myofascial pain syndromes . . . The answer to the question, 'How long will the beneficial results of specific myofascial therapy last?', depends largely on what perpetuating factors remain unresolved . . . One may view perpetuating factors also as predisposing factors, since their presence tends to make the muscles more susceptible to the activation of [trigger points] . . . Usually, one stress activates the [trigger point], then other factors perpetuate it. In some patients, these perpetuating factors are so important that their elimination results in complete relief of the pain without any local treatment."   ~~ *Doctors Janet Travell and David G. Simons*

There is much more to "Neuromuscular Therapy" or "Trigger Point Therapy" than learning referral patterns and how to search for trigger points; it is very important for a health care provider to identify and figure out *with* the patient what is causing and perpetuating their symptoms. This requires getting a complete medical history and evaluating for any potential perpetuating factors.

Trigger points are a *symptom*, not a *cause*. Needling or applying pressure to the trigger points treats the acute part of the problem, but does not resolve the underlying factors. If you get temporary relief from trigger point therapy but symptoms quickly recur, then trigger points are definitely a factor, but perpetuating factors need to be addressed in order to gain lasting relief.

This appendix will outline some general causes of trigger point activation and how to address the factors, and each muscle chapter will specifically address issues particularly pertinent to that muscle. I recommend you read all of the perpetuating factors, since you likely have more than one factor that you may not have recognized up to this point.

Acute or Chronic Viral, Bacterial, and Parasitic Infections

Acute infections, such as **colds, flu, strep throat, and bronchitis** will aggravate trigger points, particularly in a person with fibromyalgia or chronic fatigue. It is important to head off illness at the first sign in order to avoid perpetuating trigger points. When you start to get sick, take the Chinese herbs Gan Mao Ling or Yin Chiao, Echinacea, and/or homeopathics such as Osillococcinum or other appropriate homeopathics for colds, flu, or sinusitis. Once you are past the initial stage of illness, if symptoms progress, the Chinese herbs you take will be determined by your particular set of symptoms, so at this point you may need professional help to determine the proper herbs. You should have the above-mentioned herbs and homeopathics available at home so you can treat your symptoms as soon as you notice the first signs. This is particularly important if you have fibromyalgia, sinusitis, asthma, or other recurrent infections, since your trigger points will be activated by illness, and getting sick can set you back by weeks in your treatment and healing.

Outbreaks of **chronic infections**, such as **herpes simplex** (cold sores, genital herpes, herpes zoster) will also aggravate trigger points, and may need to be managed if recurrence is frequent. There are many pharmaceutical drugs and natural supplements/herbs for treating recurrent herpes infections, and some will work better than others for you. Also, if you are getting recurrent outbreaks you will want figure out what is stressing your immune system, such as allergies or emotional stress. Sometimes a herpes outbreak is the first sign you are fighting an acute illness, so that is the time to take the above-mentioned supplements.

Other chronic infections such as **sinus infections, an abscessed or impacted tooth, or urinary tract infections** will perpetuate trigger points. If you suspect a **tooth**, you will need to see your dentist for evaluation. **Urinary tract infections** (UTI's) need to be dealt with promptly. You may use over-the-counter western drugs, Chinese herbs, and cranberry (don't use sweetened juice), but if you don't respond to treatment immediately you will need to see your health care provider, since UTI's can turn into life-threatening kidney infections. Any mechanical reasons for **sinus infections** need to be dealt with for lasting relief. Naturopathic doctors can use a small inflatable balloon to open up the passages. You may need surgical intervention if the blockage is severe enough. Many people report success using a Neti Pot (get it at your health food store) to flush the sinuses with a warm saline solution. With both sinus infections and UTI's, antibiotics often won't kill all of the pathogens, and you may get a lingering, recurrent infection. However, antibiotics also work quickly, so I often recommend to patients that they combine antibiotics, acupuncture, herbs, and homeopathics to knock the infection out as quickly and completely as possible so it doesn't become a chronic problem.

The fish tapeworm, giardia, and occasionally amoeba are the most likely **parasites** to perpetuate trigger points. The fish tapeworm and giardia scar the lining of the intestine and impair your ability to absorb nutrients, and they also consume vitamin B-12. **Amoeba** can produce toxins that are passed from the intestine into the body. **Fish tapeworms** can be transmitted from raw fish. **Giardia** is most often associated with drinking untreated water from streams, but it can also be passed by an infected person not washing their hands after a bowel movement, particularly if they are preparing food or have some other hand-to-mouth contact.

Any time you have **chronic diarrhea** it is worth testing for parasites. A cheaper alternative is just to treat with herbs like grapefruit seed extract or Pulsatilla (a Chinese herb) and see if your symptoms improve. Since these will also kill off the good intestinal flora, you will want to follow treatment with a good multi-acidophilus supplement, as you would after any antibiotic. If you have blood in your stools, you should always see your health care provider immediately to rule out serious conditions. Acupuncture and Naturopathy can help resolve chronic diarrhea from most causes.

There is substantial controversy about whether **systemic candida infections** exist, though it is now listed in the Merck Manual (a medical text of illness and disease). There is abundant information on the Web regarding this subject, so I won't go into detail. Candida is a normal intestinal flora, but can multiply beyond a normal amount and cause a variety of symptoms including muscular pain. Many people report feeling much better on an anti-candida diet, and in any case it is a pretty healthy way to eat. There are many herbal products on the market for eliminating candida, including grapefruit seed extract, oil of oregano, Echinacea, Pulsatilla, and many formulas. Again, you will want to follow any of these with a good multi-acidophilus supplement to replace the beneficial intestinal flora.

Allergies and other Environmental Stressors

Both inhaled and ingested allergens perpetuate trigger points and make them harder to treat due to the subsequent histamine release. Skin tests are useful for testing for **inhaled allergens**, and there are a few methods for testing for **food allergens**.

One of the best ways to test for **food allergens** is an elimination diet, where you eliminate all foods, add them back in one at a time, and then rotate foods. You can find instructions for this in *"Prescription for Nutritional Healing"* by Balch and Balch under "Allergies." The challenge with a rotation diet is that most people are not willing to do it, as it takes a very strict control of your diet and a careful food diary for a month. As an alternative, Balch and Balch offer a quick-test. After sitting and relaxing for a few minutes, take your pulse rate for one minute, then eat the food you are testing. Keep still for 15-20 minutes and take your pulse again. If your pulse rate has increased more than ten beats per minute, eliminate this food from your diet for one month, then re-test. Naturopathic doctors offer a blood test for food sensitivities. Food allergens and sensitivities must be eliminated, but this can become challenging when you eat at other people's homes, when dining out, or while traveling. Try to keep something you *can* have with you, so you have an alternative.

There may be some ingested substances to which you are not allergic, but can aggravate your condition anyway and should be avoided. Chinese diagnosis differentiates pain by the quality of the pain (dull, achy, sharp, shooting, stabbing, burning, moving) and what makes it better or worse (i.e., rest/activity, heat/cold/damp, etc.), and some foods will aggravate certain conditions. You can see an Oriental Medicine practitioner for an evaluation of your pain and to get dietary advice, but you can try eliminating the following foods to see if it helps: coffee and black tea (yes, even decaf!), alcohol, bananas, peanuts, dairy, greasy foods, pop, sugar, wheat, and spicy foods.

Environmental allergies must be controlled as much as possible, and if you see a specialist for a skin test to identify allergens, they will make specific suggestions based on the allergen. A good HEPA air filter will help substantially, and you will need one for each room. Make sure each unit is large enough to cover the needed square footage. Not all air filters are equal, so be sure to research your options. An ozonator will kill molds, but I do not suggest leaving one running while you or pets are in the room, even though some are made for that purpose. Get an ozonator that puts out enough ozone that you can "bomb" the room while you and your pets are gone. Bomb one room at a time and close the door so that you will get a high concentration. After a few hours, hold your breath and open the windows and let the room air out for a couple of minutes before you occupy the room again. You will smell ozone (like lightening) lingering, but the air is fine to breathe after just a few minutes, so don't be concerned.

Seasonal Affective Disorder (SAD) affects millions of people to one degree or another, particularly people living closer to the North or South poles where the daylight hours are shorter in winter. SAD causes symptoms such as depression, loss of energy, decreased activity, fatigue, sleeping up to four extra hours per night, irritability and crying spells, difficulty concentrating, carbohydrate cravings, and increased appetite and weight gain. Though SAD probably does not directly cause pain, many of these symptoms *can* contribute to pain eventually. For example, if increased activity helps reduce your pain but SAD keeps you from exercising, then the SAD needs to be treated in order to help reduce your pain. Most SAD patients improve when they get additional light in their retinas. Unless you sit right next to a window in your office, you are probably not getting enough light. You may be traveling to and from work in the dark much of the year. One solution is to make sure you get outside during daylight hours, possibly for a walk at your lunch hour. Another solution is to buy a therapeutic light box. Full-spectrum lights alone are not strong enough to be of therapeutic value, so you need to get a box with reflective materials capable of producing 10,000 LUX. You need to be within 24" of the box in most cases (the light box should come with instructions that tell you how close you need to be to get 10,000 LUX), and you need to have your eyes open and looking toward the box so you get the light in your retinas.

      Toxic metals exposure has been implicated in pain syndromes. A hair analysis obtained through a naturopathic doctor can evaluate toxic levels of chemicals and mineral levels. If you find you have high levels of toxic metals, the doctor can help you with a detox program.

Emotional Factors

      While it is important to recognize the role of stress and emotional factors in creating and perpetuating illness, unfortunately all too often patients are dismissed (or medicated) by their health care providers as "just being under stress." They depart the health care provider's office with their physical symptoms not being assessed or addressed, particularly when it comes to the symptoms of pain and depression. This seems to happen more frequently to women, but I've also had male patients who had the same experience.

      Antidepressants are often prescribed, which may possibly help with the acute symptoms, but the side-effects can add to the underlying condition causing the symptoms, and a vicious cycle ensues. If you are in pain long enough, of *course* you will begin to get fatigued and depressed. If you are depressed long enough, you will probably develop pain. Anything that has gone on long enough *will* have both components.

      One of the things I like most about Oriental Medicine and homeopathy is that both modalities assume you cannot separate the physical body from the emotions, and symptoms of both are used to develop a diagnosis, and are treated simultaneously. With acupuncture there are no side-effects, and response is usually rapid. With both homeopathy and herbs (Chinese or American) the wrong prescription or dosage can have side-effects, just as with Western prescription drugs, so it is important to consult with a trained professional.

      If you are **angry, anxious or stressed**, chances are you are holding at least some of your body parts very tense, and developing trigger points. You may be hiking your shoulders up around your neck, tightening your forearms or abdomen, or tensing your gluteal muscles (women tense their gluteal muscles more often than men). In addition to dealing with the underlying cause of emotional factors, you will have to notice when you are tensing body parts, and keep consciously relaxing them over and over again. You are re-training yourself to not tense your muscles. Bio-feedback can help with this.

      If you are experiencing an unusual desire to be alone, a disinterest in your favorite activities, a decrease in job performance, and are neglecting your appearance and hygiene, you may be suffering from **depression**. Other symptoms of depression are insomnia, loss of appetite, weight loss, impotence or a lowered libido, blurred vision, a sad mood, thoughts of suicide or death, an inability to concentrate, a poor memory, indecision, mumbled speech, and negative reactions to suggestions. No one symptom will confirm a diagnosis of depression, because there are other reasons for some of these symptoms. It is the combination of symptoms that confirms a depression diagnosis. Depression lowers your pain threshold, increases pain, and adversely affects your response to trigger point therapy. (See the section on Organ Dysfunction and Disease, **thyroid**, below, since thyroid problems can be an undiagnosed cause of depression.)

If you are angry, depressed, anxious, or stressed, you will need to address this in some manner in order to speed recovery from pain. Often people suffering from severe emotional factors, chronic fatigue and/or extreme pain lack the energy to participate in their own healing. You may have difficulty feeding yourself properly or even getting out of bed, and cannot manage even mild forms of exercise such as walking -- the very things that would help you start to feel better. You may have difficulty making it to your appointments. If this describes you, you will need to do *whatever you can* to get to the point where you can start taking better care of yourself. This may mean getting antidepressants, acupuncture, homeopathy, counseling, pain relievers, and/or doing the self-help techniques in this book. Walking and deep breathing are great tension and depression-relievers. Even walking ten minutes per day (especially outside) can be extremely beneficial. Just doing one of these things will help get you started in the right direction and improve your energy and outlook.

"Secondary Gains"

Sometimes we subconsciously get something out of being sick or in pain. For example, if you have a hard time saying "no," it is easier to excuse yourself by not feeling well, rather than having to bear the brunt of the reactions you get from people who aren't used to you refusing their requests or demands. Some people have a need to stay in pain in order to get attention. Perhaps in childhood that was the only way they could get their parent's attention and they are still using that strategy as an adult. Sometimes it's easier to focus on physical symptoms than deal with underlying anxiety and emotional problems. Some people have financial reasons for not getting well, such as disability payments or lawsuit settlements, or it may get them out of some things they don't want to do.

If you find yourself complaining about your physical symptoms but not doing anything to relieve them, you might want to ask yourself what you may be getting out of staying sick. This is not always the case, as in severe depression, but it is worth at least exploring. Chances are, if you have purchased this book, you do not have subconscious needs to stay sick or in pain, since you have already taken a step to help yourself.

Good Sport Syndrome

Many people believe in pushing through the pain -- that it will make them stronger and is beneficial. Wrong! This just aggravates existing problems and makes them harder to treat. Exercise should be comfortable, such as alternating running with walking or resting in between weight repetitions, and using weights that aren't too heavy. If you tend to overdo things, you will need to back off on your activities and add them back in slowly with the guidance of your practitioner. Returning to activities too soon or excessively will quickly wipe out your therapeutic progress.

Injuries

A healthy muscle is pliable to the touch when it is not being used, but will feel firm if called upon for action. If a muscle feels firm at rest, it is tight in an unhealthy way (even if you work-out). I like to use an analogy of a rubber band or stick. Imagine that a sudden, unexpected force is applied to the "stick," or tight muscle (such as a fall). Like a stick, the muscle will be damaged. If a sudden force is applied to a pliable muscle, or "rubberband," it will stretch with the force instead, and will be much less likely to be injured. Since latent trigger points restrict range-of-motion to some degree, and almost everyone has some latent trigger points, a muscle may be tight and restricted without you being aware of it, and can be easily injured if a sudden force is applied.

Injuries are one of the most common initiators of trigger points. **People who exercise regularly are less likely to develop trigger points** than those who exercise occasionally and overdo it. If you have an injury, begin treatment as soon as possible. Apply cold during the first 48 hours, and use some form of arnica homeopathic orally and/or topically as soon as possible. There are Chinese herb formulas for trauma that you can get from an acupuncturist or possibly a health food store. Have these available in your medicine cabinet since it may be hard for you to go to the store after you are injured, and because these work best when started immediately after the injury. See an acupuncturist or massage therapist who is experienced in working with recent injuries. You may also need to see a chiropractor, osteopathic physician, or physical therapist.

Surgeries will likely leave some amount of scar tissue, which can perpetuate trigger points in adjacent muscle fibers. **Scar tissue** can be broken up to an extent with cross-friction massage. Because this is usually fairly painful, I only work on scars for a few minutes each appointment, and I warn the patient that it will be painful but that I won't do it for more than a few minutes. Most patients will not work on their own scars vigorously enough due to the pain level. Acupuncture can treat scar tissue and help eliminate the pain from trigger points around the area. I recommend using both cross-friction massage and acupuncture as part of the treatment protocol, rather than just one or the other.

Mechanical Stresses

Chronic mechanical stresses are one of the most common causes of trigger point activation and perpetuation, and are nearly always correctable. A **skeletal asymmetry**, including an anatomically shorter leg and a small hemipelvis (either the right or left half of the pelvis) can be corrected with shoe lifts and butt lifts. [NOTE: In this book, reference to a "shorter leg" refers to a *true* anatomical leg length inequality where the bones are shorter on one side, rather than the "shorter leg" caused by a spinal mis-alignment, which is a term chiropractors use.] A **skeletal disproportion**, such as a long second toe can be corrected with shoe orthotics, and short upper arms can be corrected with ergonomically correct furniture. Vertebral subluxation and other bones-out-alignment can be adjusted by a chiropractor or osteopathic physician, especially if the muscles are also first relaxed by an acupuncturist or massage therapist. Your physical therapist may be trained in manipulations.

Wearing appropriate shoes can help relieve symptoms in your entire body (see "Abuse of Muscles," below). **Orthotics** can help even more. My favorite non-corrective orthotics are the Superfeet brand. They have a deep heel cup which helps prevent pronation (more weight on the inside of your foot) and supination (more weight on the outside of the foot), and they have excellent arch support. Superfeet has a variety of models, including cheaper non-custom "Trim-to-Fit" footbeds, and moderately-priced custom molded footbeds to provide support in a variety of footwear. See Superfeet.com to learn more about their products. If you find you need corrective orthotics, you will need to see a podiatrist. If you decide to get custom orthotics, be sure to work on your trigger points first, because as the muscles relax you will stand differently and the orthotics need to be formed for the corrected stance.

Misfitting furniture is a major cause of muscular pain, particularly in the work place. There are companies that specialize in coming into your work place and correcting your office arrangement, and fitting you for furniture that fits your body. Your employer may balk at the cost, but if they don't change your misfitting furniture, they will end up paying for it in lost work time and worker's compensation claims.

I see a lot of what I call "mouse injuries" -- arm and shoulder pain due to using a computer mouse for extended periods of time without proper arm support. The keyboard should be kept as close to lap level as possible. When not using your computer, your elbows and forearms should rest evenly on either your work surface or armrests of the proper height. Your computer screen should be directly in front of you with the middle of the screen slightly below eye level, and the copy attached to the side of the screen, so that you may look directly forward as much as possible. Your knees should fit under your desk, and the chair needs to be close enough that you can lean against your backrest. A good chair will have a backrest with a slope of 25 to 30-degrees back from the vertical which supports both the lumbar area and the mid-back. The seat should be low enough that your feet rest flat on the floor without compression of the thigh by the front edge of the seat, high enough that not all the pressure is put on the buttocks, and slightly hollowed out to accommodate the buttocks. The armrests must be high enough to provide support for the elbows without having to lean to the side, but not so high as to cause the shoulders to hike up. The upholstery needs to be firm and casters should be avoided. I highly recommend headsets for phones to solve neck and back pain.

A lumbar support helps correct round-shouldered posture. Most chiropractic offices carry lumbar supports of varying thickness. I recommend getting one for the car (most car seats actually *curve the wrong way* in the lumbar area) and your favorite seat at home, and investing in a good chair for the office, even if your employer won't. Try to avoid sitting in or on anything without back support, which causes you to sit with your shoulders and upper back slumped forward. When going to sporting events, picnics, or other places you won't have a back support, bring a *Crazy Creek Chair*™ (or something similar) to provide at least some support. You can get one through most of the major sporting goods suppliers for about $49, a good investment in your back, and they are very lightweight for carrying. Or consider a lightweight collapsible chair, also available at sporting goods stores.

Sleeping in a sagging bed can cause back and hip problems. (See the section on Sleep Problems below).

But properly fitting furniture won't help as much if you are not also conscientious of avoiding **poor posture**. If you slouch at your desk or on your couch at home, or read in bed, for example, your muscles will suffer. **Abuse of muscles** includes poor body mechanics (i.e., lifting improperly), long periods of immobility (i.e., sitting at a desk without a break), repetitive movements (i.e., computer use), holding your body in an awkward position for long periods (i.e., dentists and mechanics), and excessively quick and jerky movements (i.e., sports). Learn to lift properly and take frequent breaks from anything you must do for long time periods.

If you have a habit of immobilizing your muscles to protect against pain, you will need to start gently increasing your range of motion as you inactivate trigger points. Don't keep stressing the muscles to see if it still hurts or to demonstrate to your treating professionals where you have to move it to in order to get it to hurt -- if you keep repeating this motion, you will just keep the trigger points activated.

Be sure to sit while putting clothing on your lower body. Don't wear high heels or cowboy boots. If you carry a purse, get a strap long enough that you can wear it diagonally across your body, rather than over one shoulder. If you use a day pack, put the straps over both shoulders. Without realizing it, you are hiking up one shoulder at least a little to keep the straps from slipping off no matter *how* light your purse or pack may be. Notice whether you hold your shoulders up or are tightening muscles such as your butt, arms, or abdomen when you are under stress. You will need to re-train yourself to break this habit.

If you are clenching your jaw or grinding your teeth, see a dentist for help. The soft plastic bite splints found over-the-counter in pharmacies are too soft and do not help temporomandibular joint dysfunction. You need to be fitted by your dentist for a hard, slippery acrylic night guard.

Constricting clothing can lead to muscular problems. My rule of thumb is, if the clothing item leaves an elastic mark or indentation in the skin, it is too tight and is cutting off proper circulation. Check your bras, socks, ties, and belts to see if they are too tight.

Be sure to check muscles listed in the muscle chapters that can cause "satellite trigger points," since this is one perpetuating cause. For example, if you find trigger points in the abdominal muscles but trigger points quickly recur, check the paraspinal muscles also, because trigger points there can refer to the abdominal area and cause trigger points to be reactivated.

Nutritional Problems and Diet

Doctors Travell and Simons found that almost half of their patients required treatment for **vitamin inadequacies** to obtain lasting relief from the pain and dysfunction of trigger points, and thought it was one of the most important perpetuating factors to address. They found **the most important were the water-soluble vitamins B-1, B-6, B-12, folic acid, vitamin C, and the minerals calcium, magnesium, iron and potassium**. Other researchers have now added **vitamin D** to that list.

The more deficient in nutrients you are, the more symptoms you will have, and your trigger points and nervous system will be more hyper-irritable. Even if a blood test determines you are at the low end of the normal range, you may still need more of a nutrient, since your body will pull nutrients from the tissues before it will allow a decrease in the blood levels. Several factors may lead to nutrient insufficiency:

- An inadequate intake of a nutrient
- Impaired nutrient absorption
- Inadequate nutrient utilization
- An increased need by the body
- A nutrient leaving the body too quickly
- A nutrient being destroyed within the body too quickly

You may be in a **high risk group** if you are: elderly, pregnant or nursing, an alcoholic or other drug user, poor, depressed, or seriously ill. If you tend to diet by leaving out important food groups, or have an eating disorder, you will also deplete yourself of necessary nutrients.

- Even if you have a fairly healthy diet, because our soils have been depleted in nutrients from too frequent crop-rotations, chemical fertilizers, and long shipping distances, our food does not provide all the nutrition we require. In addition, many of us don't have a very balanced diet, and processed foods do not contain as much nutrition as fresh-prepared. Most people need to take some kind of **multi-supplement** to ensure proper nutrition, especially if you fall into one of the high risk groups mentioned above. Because some vitamins require the presence of other vitamins, a good multi-supplement ensures the needed combination is present. Be sure to check the label to make sure there are adequate minerals in a multi -- you may need to also take a multi-mineral. Improving your nutrient intake to see if it improves your symptoms is an easy and relatively inexpensive therapy to try. Take your vitamins with food, since some need to bind with substances found in food in order to be absorbed.

   Building up sufficient levels of vitamin B-12, vitamin D, and iron may take several months; don't get discouraged if you don't see immediate results, though you may start gradually feeling better within a few weeks from taking multivitamin and multimineral supplements.

- You may still need to be tested by a health care provider for inadequacies, since some people are not able to absorb certain nutrients, and need to have them injected or mega-dosed. For example, some people cannot absorb B-12, and need to get intramuscular injections to provide that necessary vitamin.

- **Take your vitamins and herbs when you are *not* sick** -- the germs also like the vitamins and herbs and they will get stronger. See the section above on Acute or Chronic Viral, Bacterial, and Parasitic Infections for suggestions on how to head off illness. Once all symptoms have abated, you may switch back to your regular vitamins and herbs.

- How well your **digestive system** is functioning is also a factor. If you are not digesting well, you do not have enough enzymes or possibly hydrochloric acid to break down food properly. Taking digestive enzymes or hydrochloric acid for long periods is not a good solution, because they will take over the natural function of your body. Supplementation can be used in the short term, but you need to repair the body's natural function so it can perform its own job properly. **Digestive problems** can be addressed with the help of an acupuncturist, herbalist, or naturopath. They can give you dietary recommendations based on your unique set of health problems and constitution, and prescribe herbs to re-balance your systems.

- It is a common mis-conception that raw foods and whole grains are the healthiest way to eat. It is actually better to **cook your food** (not overcook!) in order to start the chemical breakdown process, so your digestive system doesn't have to work as hard. If you are having trouble digesting, white rice and bread are easier to digest than whole grains. Soups are nutritious and easy to digest.

- **Fasting** is hard on the digestive system. If you want to do a cleanse, use herbs and psyllium, but don't stop eating.

- Most people should not be strict vegetarians. At the very least you should eat organic eggs for a **high-quality protein** source. Most vegetarians are not very good about combining foods, and even if they are, most still seem to feel better when they add high-quality animal protein back into their diet. Plant sources contain mainly the pyridoxol form of B-6, but animal sources contain both the pyridoxal and pyridoxamine forms of B-6, and are less susceptible to the loss of the vitamin due to cooking or preserving. B-12 is *only* found in animal proteins, including dairy products. Brewer's yeast does not contain B-12, unless the yeast is grown on a special B-12-containing substrate.

- If you have **chronic diarrhea**, you will not retain food long enough in the intestines to absorb nutrients. You will need to identify and eliminate the source of diarrhea. Acupuncture, herbs, and dietary changes can often successfully address this problem.

- Excess **caffeine** increases muscle tension and trigger point irritability, leading to increased pain. Dr.'s Travell and Simons state that "... caffeine has long been known to cause a persistent contracture, or caffeine rigor, of muscle fibers. This rigor is due to enhancement by caffeine of the release of calcium from the sarcoplasmic reticulum and to interference with the rebinding of calcium ions by the sarcoplasmic reticulum." They found that caffeine in excess of 150 mg daily (more than two eight-ounce cups of regular coffee) would lead to caffeine rigor. Based on my clinical experience, some people can't even consume 150 mg without aggravating their pain. In counting your daily intake, be sure to count any caffeine in the drugs you are taking, and remember that espresso and similar drinks will have far greater amounts of caffeine. There are websites that list caffeine amounts for foods and beverages.

- **Alcohol** aggravates trigger points by decreasing serum and tissue folate levels. It increases the body's need for vitamin C, while decreasing the body's ability to absorb it. **Tobacco** also increases the need for vitamin C. In Chinese Medicine, caffeine and alcohol are said to be very "qi stagnating." **Marijuana** is very stagnating also, and stays in your system for about three months after smoking it. Stagnation is one cause of pain, therefore using any of the above substances will increase your pain level.

- Eliminating foods and beverages that aggravate your condition (such as allergins, coffee, and alcohol) may not be enough, if the underlying condition that was caused by the food has not been resolved. For example, if you have been eating damp-producing foods (like dairy and peanut butter) which has led to dampness in the muscles (as in fibromyalgia), even if you stop ingesting the food or beverage you still have dampness in the muscles that must be eliminated. Plan on avoiding the necessary foods for two months minimum *in conjunction* with acupuncture and/or herbs and other supplements, in order to determine whether eliminating the food is helpful. Many people will stop ingesting a food or drink for one week, decide it hasn't made a difference, and then re-start their regular diet. Or the food or beverage is so important to them that they'd rather have pain and other medical conditions, than give the substance up. Reaching a conclusion after one week is one way to justify continuing to ingest the substance.

- **Herbs** should be taken with the advice of a qualified practitioner. I've seen many people who have injured their digestive systems by taking too many herbs, or herbs that are improper for their conditions and constitution. What may be the correct herb for a friend or a family member may not be the correct herb for you, so seek professional advice.

- Room-temperature **water** is better than cold drinks -- if you drink something cold, your stomach has to work harder to warm it up, and it taxes the digestive system. Drink about two quarts per day, or more if you have a larger body mass or sweat a lot. A general rule of thumb for kids and adults weighing more than 100 pounds is your body weight multiplied by the number of ounces (i.e., 140 lbs. = 70 ounces). Drink at least one extra quart per day if it is very hot out, and extra water during and immediately after a work-out. If you drink *too* much water, you can deplete Vitamin B-1 (thiamine). Thirst is not necessarily a good indicator of whether or not you are dehydrated. Your urine should be a light yellow, unless you have just taken a multivitamin or B-vitamin supplement.

- **Don't drink distilled water**, because you need the minerals found in non-distilled water. If you drink bottled water, make sure you know its source, and that it is not distilled. This industry is not currently regulated, so you may need to do some research on the company.

Vitamins

- **Vitamin C** reduces post-exercise soreness and corrects the capillary fragility which leads to easy bruising. (Hint: if you don't remember how you got a bruise, you are likely bruising too easily.) It is essential for collagen formation (connective tissue) and forming bones. Vitamin C is required for synthesis of the neurotransmitters norepinephrine and serotonin, is needed for your body's response to stress, is important for immune system function, and decreases the irritability of trigger points caused by infection.
Too *much* Vitamin C can lead to watery diarrhea or non-specific urethritis. However, Vitamin C helps terminate diarrhea due to food allergies. Vitamin C daily doses above 400mg are not used by the body, and 1000mg/day increases the risk of kidney stone formation, so mega-dosing with Vitamin C is not necessary nor recommended. Women taking estrogen or oral contraceptives may need 500mg/day.

Vitamin C is likely to be deficient in smokers, alcoholics, older people (the presence of Vitamin C in the tissues decreases with age), infants fed primarily on cows' milk (usually between the ages of 6-12 months), people with chronic diarrhea, psychiatric patients, and fad dieters. Initial symptoms of deficiency include weakness, lethargy, irritability, vague aching pains in the joints and muscles, easy bruising, and possibly weight loss. In severe cases of Vitamin C deficiency (scurvy), the gums become red, swollen, bleed easily, and teeth may become loose and fall out.

Do not take Vitamin C with antacids; since Vitamin C is ascorbic acid, and the purpose of an antacid is to neutralize acid, antacids will neutralize Vitamin C and make it ineffective. Food sources include citrus fruits and *fresh* juices, *raw* broccoli, *raw* Brussels sprouts, collard, kale, turnip greens, guava, *raw* sweet peppers, cabbage, and potatoes

- **Taking too many vitamins A, D, and E, and folic acid** can cause symptoms similar to deficiencies, so don't mega-dose on those supplements unless a health care provider has determined your condition warrants it.

- **Thiamine (Vitamin B-1)** is essential for normal nerve function and energy production within muscle cells. Diminished pain and temperature sensitivity and an inability to detect vibrations indicate you are low in thiamine. You may also possibly experience calf cramping at night, slight sweating, constipation, and fatigue. B-1 is needed for proper thyroid hormone levels (see the section on Organ Dysfunction and Disease below). Abuse of alcohol reduces thiamine absorption, and absorption is further reduced if liver disease is also present. The tannin in black tea, antacid use, and a magnesium deficiency can also prevent the absorption of thiamine. Thiamine can be destroyed by processing foods, and by heating them to temperatures above 212º F (100º C). Thiamine is excreted too rapidly when taking diuretics or drinking too much water. Lean pork, kidney, liver, beef, eggs, fish, beans, nuts, and some whole grain cereals (if the hull and germ are present) are good sources of thiamine.

- **Pyridoxine (Vitamin B-6)** is important for nerve function, energy metabolism, amino acid metabolism, and synthesis of neurotransmitters including norepinephrine and serotonin, which strongly influence pain perception. Deficiency of B-6 results in anemia, reduced absorption and storage of B-12, increased excretion of Vitamin C, blocked synthesis of niacin, and can lead to a hormonal imbalance. Deficiency of B-6 will manifest as symptoms of one of the other B-vitamins, since B-6 is needed in order for all the others to perform their functions. The need for B-6 increases with age and increased protein consumption. Tropical sprue and alcohol use interfere with its absorption. Use of **oral contraceptives** increases your requirement for B-6, and impairs glucose tolerance. This can lead to depression if you don't supplement with B-6, particularly if you already have a history of depression. Corticosteroid use, excessive alcohol use, pregnancy and lactation, antitubercular drugs, uremia, and hyperthyroidism also increase the need for B-6. Sources of B-6 include liver, kidney, chicken (white meat), halibut, tuna, English walnuts, soybean flour, navy beans, bananas, and avocados. There is also some amount of B-6 present in yeast, lean beef, egg yolk, and whole wheat.

- **Cobalamin (Vitamin B-12) and Folic Acid** need to be taken together to form erythrocytes (a type of red blood cell) and rapidly dividing cells such as those found in the gastrointestinal tract, and for fatty acid synthesis used in the formation of parts of certain nerve fibers. B-12 is needed for both fat and carbohydrate metabolism. A deficiency can result in **pernicious (megaloblastic) anemia**, which reduces oxygen coming to the site of the trigger point, adding to the dysfunctional cycle and increasing pain. A deficiency of B-12 may also cause symptoms such as non-specific depression, fatigue, an exaggerated startle reaction to noise or touch, and an increased susceptibility to trigger points. B-12 is only found in animal products or supplements. Several drugs may impair the absorption of B-12, as can mega-doses of Vitamin C for long periods of time.

- A **folate deficiency** (also known as **folic acid** when in the synthetic form) can cause you to be fatigued easily, sleep poorly, and feel discouraged and depressed. It can cause "restless legs," diffuse muscular pain, diarrhea, a loss of sensation in the extremities, and you may feel cold frequently, along with a slightly lower basal body temperature than the "normal" 98.6º F (37º C). Folic acid deficiency is very prevalent and can lead to **megaloblastic anemia**. In the U.S., studies have shown that at least 15% of Caucasians are deficient, while at least 30% of African-Americans and Latinos are deficient. At least half of Canadians eat less than the dietary recommendation. Part of the problem is that 50-95% of the folate content of foods may be destroyed in food processing and preparation, so even if you eat folate sources, you may not be receiving the benefit. A necessary conversion in the digestive system is inhibited by peas, beans, citrus fruits, acidic foods, and antacids, so eat these separately from your folic acid sources. The best sources of folate are leafy vegetables, yeast, organ meat, fruit, and lightly cooked vegetables such as broccoli and asparagus. You are at greatest risk for folate deficiency if you are elderly, have a bowel disorder, are pregnant or lactating, or use drugs and alcohol regularly. Certain other drugs will also deplete folate, such as anti-inflammatories (including aspirin), diuretics, estrogens (such as birth control pills), and anti-convulsants. You must also have adequate B-12 intake in order to absorb folic acid, plus only taking one of these can mask a severe deficiency in the other.

- **Vitamin D** is required for both the absorption and the utilization of calcium and phosphorus. It is necessary for growth and thyroid function, it protects against muscle weakness, and helps regulate the heartbeat. It is important for the prevention of cancer, osteoarthritis, osteoporosis, and calcium deficiency. A mild deficiency of vitamin D may manifest as a loss of appetite, a burning sensation in the mouth and throat, diarrhea, insomnia, visual problems, and weight loss. It has been estimated that close to 90% of patients with chronic musculoskeletal pain may have a vitamin D deficiency.

  Vitamin D-3 is synthesized by the skin when exposed to the sun's UV rays. Unfortunately, many people don't get enough sun exposure, especially if they live at latitudes or in climates with little sun available during the winter months. Exposing your face and arms to the sun for 15 minutes three times per week will ensure that your body synthesizes an adequate amount of vitamin D. Because the amount of exposure needed varies from person to person and also depends on geographical location, you will need to do some personal research and perhaps consult with a dermatologist to determine the proper amount for you. Food sources of vitamin D include salmon, halibut, sardines, tuna, and eggs. Other sources include dairy products, dandelion greens, liver, oatmeal, and sweet potatoes. If you take supplements, look for the D-3 form, or fish oil capsules.

Minerals

Inadequate salt, calcium/magnesium, or potassium can lead to **muscle cramping**.

- Do not entirely eliminate **salt** from your diet, especially if you sweat. You do need some salt in your diet (unless you have been instructed otherwise by your health care provider for certain medical conditions), though you don't want to overdo it either.

- **Calcium, magnesium, potassium, and iron** are needed for proper muscle function. Iron is required for oxygen transport to the muscle fibers. Calcium is essential for releasing acetylcholine at the nerve terminal, and both calcium and magnesium are needed for the contracting mechanism of the muscle fiber. Potassium is needed to get the muscle fiber quickly ready for its next contraction. Deficiency of these minerals increases the irritability of trigger points. Calcium, magnesium, and potassium should be taken together, because an increase in one can deplete the others. Also needed for good health but not as important for muscle function are zinc, iodine, copper, manganese, chromium, selenium, and molybdenum.

  It is especially important to take **calcium** for at least a few years prior to menopause to help prevent osteoporosis. Vitamin D is needed for calcium uptake. Food sources of calcium include dairy (though this is not recommended for people with damp conditions, such as fibromyalgia), salmon, sardines, seafood, green leafy vegetables, almonds, asparagus, blackstrap molasses, brewer's yeast, broccoli, cabbage, carob, collards, dandelion greens, figs, filberts, kale, kelp, mustard greens, oats, parsley, prunes, sesame seeds, tofu, turnip greens, and whey.

- Do not take Tums or other **antacids** as a source of **calcium**. Stomach acid is needed for the uptake of calcium, but an antacid neutralizes stomach acid. So even if there is calcium present, it cannot be used. If you must take an antacid, take it several hours apart from your calcium/magnesium supplement so you will maximize your mineral uptake. **Calcium channel blockers** prescribed for high blood pressure inhibit the uptake of calcium into the sarcoplasmic reticulum of vascular smooth muscles and cardiac muscles. Since this is likely also true for skeletal muscles, calcium channel blockers would also make trigger points worse, and more difficult to treat. See your health care provider to find out if you can switch to a different medication. Consider treating the underlying causes of hypertension with acupuncture, diet changes, exercise, or whatever is appropriate to your particular set of circumstances.

- **Magnesium deficiency** is less likely to occur as a result of an inadequate dietary intake in a healthy diet as it is to malabsorption, malnutrition, kidney disease, or fluid and electrolyte loss. Magnesium is depleted after strenuous physical exercise, but proper amounts of exercise coupled with an adequate intake of magnesium improves the efficiency of cellular metabolism and improves cardio-respiratory performance. Consumption of alcohol, the use of diuretics, chronic diarrhea, consumption of fluoride, and high amounts of zinc and Vitamin D increase the body's need for magnesium.

  Magnesium is found in most foods, especially dairy products (though this is not recommended for people with damp conditions, such as fibromyalgia), fish, meat, seafood, apples, apricots, avocados, bananas, blackstrap molasses, brewer's yeast, brown rice, figs, garlic, kelp, lima beans, millet, nuts, peaches, black-eyes peas, salmon, sesame seeds, tofu, green leafy vegetable, wheat, and whole grains.

- A diet high in fats, refined sugars, and too much salt causes **potassium deficiency**, as does the use of laxatives and some diuretics. Diarrhea will also deplete potassium. If you suffer from urinary frequency, particularly if your urine is clear rather than light yellow, try taking potassium. Frequent urination causes potassium deficiency, and potassium deficiency may cause frequent urination, and a cycle of depletion ensues. Food sources of potassium include fruit (especially bananas and citrus fruits), potatoes, green leafy vegetables, wheat germ, beans, lentils, nuts, dates, and prunes.

- **Iron deficiency** can lead to **anemia**, and is usually caused by excessive blood loss from a heavy menses, hemorrhoids, intestinal bleeding, donating blood too often, or ulcers. Iron deficiency can also be caused by a long-term illness, prolonged use of antacids, poor digestion, excess coffee or black tea consumption, or the chronic use of NSAID's (non-steroidal anti-inflammatory drugs, such as ibuprofen). Calcium in milk, cheese, or as a supplement can impair absorption of iron, therefore you should take your calcium supplement separately. Do not take an iron supplement if you have an infection or cancer. The body stores it in order to withhold it from bacteria, and in the case of cancer, it may suppress the cancer-killing function of certain cells.

  Early symptoms of iron deficiency include impaired work performance, fatigue, reduced endurance, and an inability to stay warm when exposed to a moderately cold environment. 9-11% of menstruating females in the U.S. are iron deficient, and the world-wide prevalence is about 15%. Iron is best absorbed with Vitamin C. Generally food sources are adequate for improving iron levels for most people. Good sources of iron include eggs, fish, liver, meat, poultry, green leafy vegetables, whole grains, almonds, avocados, beets, blackstrap molasses, brewer's yeast, dates, egg yolks, kelp, kidney and lima beans, lentils, millet, parsley, peaches, pears, dried prunes, pumpkin, raisins, rice and wheat bran, sesame seeds, and soybeans.

One of my favorite books is "*Prescription for Nutritional Healing*" by James F. Balch, M.D., and Phyllis A. Balch, C.N.C.. It has a comprehensive list of vitamins, minerals, amino acids, antioxidants, and enzymes, and food sources for each. It has sections on common disorders listing supplements needed to treat each condition, and helpful hints.

Hormonal Changes

Women are more likely than men to develop trigger points. I have noticed this is particularly true in **menopausal** women. Some teenagers (of both sexes) going through **puberty** also seem to have a tendency to develop trigger points, leading me to believe there is a connection between hormonal changes and one potential cause of trigger points.

Organ Dysfunction and Disease

Thyroid

Both **thyroid inadequacy** (also known as hypometabolism or subclinical hypothyroidism) and **hypothyroidism** will cause and perpetuate trigger points. Hypothyroid patients may experience early morning stiffness, and pain and weakness of the shoulder girdle. Both thyroid inadequacy and hypothyroidism will produce symptoms of cold (and sometimes heat) intolerance, cold hands and feet, muscle aches and pains especially with cold rainy weather, constipation, menstrual problems, weight gain, dry skin, and fatigue and lethargy. Muscles feel rather hard to the touch, and even if a patient is on a thyroid supplement, I've noticed they are still somewhat prone to trigger points, since it is hard to fine-tune the medication exactly to the amount your body would produce if you still had a healthy thyroid organ. Some studies report the prevalence of subclinical hypothyroidism to be as high as 17% in women and 7% in men. Occasionally patients with inadequate metabolism may be thin, nervous, and hyperactive, which may result in a health care provider failing to consider subclinical hypothyroidism.

Patients with low thyroid function may be **low in thiamine (Vitamin B-1)**. Before starting on thyroid medication, try supplementing with thiamine to see if that corrects your thyroid hormone levels. If you are already on thyroid medication and you start taking B-1, you may start exhibiting symptoms of *hyper*thyroidism, and your medication dosage needs to be adjusted. If you are low in B-1 at the time of starting thyroid medication, you may develop symptoms of acute thiamine deficiency, which may be misinterpreted as an intolerance to the medication. After the B-1 deficiency is corrected, you will likely tolerate the medication. You will need to supplement with B-1 prior to and during thyroid hormone therapy to avoid a deficiency. Total body potassium is low in hypothyroidism, and high in hyperthyroidism, so you may need to adjust your potassium intake also.

Smoking impairs the action of thyroid hormone and will make any related symptoms worse. Several pharmaceutical drugs can also affect thyroid hormone levels, such as lithium, anti-convulsants, those that contain iodine, and glucocorticoid steroids, so check with your pharmacist if you have been diagnosed with hypothyroidism and are taking another medication.

A simple **home test** to check your thyroid function is to place a thermometer in your armpit for 10 minutes upon waking but before getting out of bed. Normal underarm temperature for men and post-menopausal women is 98º F (36.7º C). If you are still menstruating your temperature should be around 97.5º F (36.4º C) prior to ovulation, and 98.5º F (36.9º C) following ovulation. If your temperature is lower than this, you will want to check with your health care provider. Often health care providers will only initially test the TSH level, which may still be normal if you have hypometabolism rather than hypothyroidism. A radioimmunoassay measures T3 and T4 levels, and gives a more complete picture of the thyroid function.

If you are suffering from depression, be sure to insist that your thyroid levels are tested before starting on anti-depressant medication. I've had more than one patient (especially men) where hypothyroidism was discovered only after they had been medicated for some time.

Hypoglycemia

Both **postprandial (reactive) and fasting hypoglycemia** cause and perpetuate trigger points, and make trigger points more difficult to treat. Symptoms of both are sweating, trembling and shakiness, increased heart rate, and anxiety. Activation of trigger points in the *sternocleidomastoid* muscle by a hypoglycemic reaction may lead to dizziness and headaches. If allowed to progress, symptoms can include visual disturbances, restlessness, and impaired speech and thinking. Missing or delaying a meal does not cause hypoglycemia in a healthy person. A hypoglycemic reaction to a delayed meal usually indicates a problem with the liver, adrenal glands, or pituitary gland. Postprandial hypoglycemia usually occurs two to three hours after eating a meal rich in carbohydrates, and is most like to occur when you are under high stress.

Causes will need to be identified and addressed, if possible. Symptoms will be relieved by eating smaller, more frequent meals with fewer carbohydrates, more protein, and some fat. Avoid all caffeine, alcohol, and tobacco (even second-hand smoke). If you are waking with headaches or pain or having trouble sleeping, try eating a small snack or drink a little juice before bedtime to see if it relieves your symptoms; it usually helps. Acupuncture is quite successful in stabilizing blood sugar.

Gout

Gout will aggravate trigger points and make them difficult to treat. Doctors Travell and Simons recommend keeping the gout under control and taking Vitamin C, and then subsequent treatment of trigger points will be more effective.

Sleep Problems

Pain can interrupt sleep, and interrupted sleep can perpetuate trigger points. It is useful to know whether your sleep was interrupted before your pain started, or whether your sleep was sound and restful. If your sleep was poor prior to the pain, then there is another underlying factor which needs to be addressed to help solve the problem.

Be sure you are not sleeping poorly due to being **too warm or too cold**. If you have **problems falling asleep**, try improving your nutrition and your water intake first. Take a calcium/magnesium supplement before bedtime. If you are **waking easily due to noise**, try Mack's™ soft silicon earplugs (my favorite), and try breathing deeply until you fall back to sleep. If you can't stop thinking, you sleep lightly and wake frequently, you wake early and can't fall back to sleep, are menopausal, and/or have vivid and disturbing dreams, try acupuncture and Chinese herbs.

Even if you only drink **caffeine** in the morning, it still disturbs your nighttime sleep pattern, as does **alcohol**. If you choose to give up caffeine, it will take about two weeks before your energy starts to even out and you don't feel like you have to use it to get going in the morning. **Computer use in the evening** stimulates the brain and makes it hard to fall asleep and sleep restfully. If **urinary frequency** is disturbing your sleep, try acupuncture and herbs, and increasing your potassium intake.

Consider whether your **adrenal glands** could be excreting too much cortisol (the "stress hormone"). If you are continually stressed, or if you are pushing yourself too hard and push through fatigue instead of resting or taking a nap, you will excrete more cortisol and have more difficulty sleeping at night. A Naturopathic doctor can administer a saliva test for adrenal function.

Make sure you are not being exposed to **allergens** at night. Get inexpensive soft plastic covers for your pillows and mattress, since many people are allergic to mites, and they live in your bedding. If you have a down comforter or pillow, you may be allergic to the feathers, even if you are not exhibiting classic allergic symptoms, such as sneezing and itchy eyes.

Beds that are too soft can cause a lot of muscular problems, and you may not know it is too soft. Patients usually insist their mattress is firm enough, but when queried further, will admit that sleeping on a mat on the floor gives them relief when the pain is particularly bad. If this is the case, your mattress is not firm enough, no matter how much money you spent on it or how well it worked for someone else. Different people have needs for different kinds of mattresses. An all-cotton futon is very firm, and may be best for some people. The "Sleep Number" bed allows you to change the firmness and some models have an option to control firmness separately for each side of the bed. A lot of people like memory foam beds, but I personally find them too soft. Try putting some camp mats on the floor and sleeping on them for a week. If you feel better, it is time for a new, firmer mattress. Mattresses really only last about five to seven years, and should then be replaced. Some furniture stores will let you try a mattress out for a time period before making a final decision. Be sure you have a **pillow** that keeps your head in line with your spine -- not too high or too low. Sleeping on the couch should definitely be avoided.

If pain disturbs you at night, I sometimes suggest to patients that they keep their self-help ball collection by their bed so that if they wake they can work on their trigger points, and hopefully fall back to sleep once the pain is reduced. The danger in this is that *you have to be sure you don't fall asleep on the ball*! It will cut off the circulation for too long, and make the trigger points worse. It is an easy thing to do when you are fatigued and in pain, and suddenly the pain is reduced or gone, so don't use the ball in bed unless you are sure you will not fall asleep on it.

Spinal Mis-alignments and Other Problems

Vertebrae may be out-of-alignment, and need to be adjusted by a chiropractor or osteopathic physician, or mobilized by a physical therapist. Usually there is also a muscular component that caused the mis-alignment to begin with, so a combined approach of skeletal mobilization and massage or acupuncture is probably necessary for lasting relief. A chiropractor or osteopathic physician will likely take x-rays at the initial visit to evaluate your spine. If you have already had x-rays taken, bring them with you to the visit so you can avoid duplicating x-rays.

Herniated and bulging disks may be very successfully treated with acupuncture (especially Plum Blossom technique), but if you don't get some relief fairly quickly, you may want to consider surgery if you have insurance. Spinal surgery has gotten so sophisticated that many surgeries are fairly minor procedures that have you back on your feet the next day. If you have **stenosis** (a narrowing of the central spinal cord canal or the holes the nerves come out of) acupuncture will help with pain, but not the stenosis, so surgery is probably the best option. With any surgery there is a certain amount of risk, so be sure to discuss this with your operating physician, and make sure you understand the procedure. If you are still unsure, get a second opinion from another surgeon. Disc problems and stenosis need to be confirmed with an MRI.

Bone spurs and narrowed disc spaces can cause pain. But in a random sample of the population you will find many people with bone spurs and narrowed disc spaces with no pain, and many people with pain and no bone spurs or narrowed disc spaces, so don't assume these are causing your problems, even if a health care provider has made this assumption.

I always start with the assumption that trigger points are at least part of the problem, if not all of the problem, and treat accordingly. If a patient doesn't receive some relief fairly quickly, then I know there may be something else going on and I refer them to someone who can evaluate them with an x-ray or MRI.

If you have had surgery and your pain continues, trigger points are the likely culprit, and need to be treated for lasting relief. If you still do not get relief, there is a possibility the pain is due to scar tissue from the surgery compressing a nerve root, so you will need to check with your health care provider.

Laboratory Tests

Laboratory tests may be necessary to help diagnose some of the systemic perpetuating factors. With blood chemistry profiles, an elevated erythrocyte sedimentation rate (**SED Rate**) may indicate a chronic bacterial infection, polymyositis, polymyalgia rheumatica, rheumatoid arthritis, or cancer. A decreased **erythrocyte count** and/or **low hemoglobin** points to anemia. A mean corpuscular volume (**MCV**) of over 92fl indicates the likelihood of a folate or B-12 deficiency. **Eosinophilia** may indicate an allergy or intestinal parasitic infection. An increase in **monocytes** can indicate low thyroid function, infectious mononucleosis, or an acute viral infection. Increased serum **cholesterol** can be caused by a problem with low thyroid function, and a low serum cholesterol can indicate folate deficiency. High **uric acid** levels indicate hyperuricemia and possibly gout.

Iron deficiency is detected by checking the **serum ferritin** level. A **fasting blood test** is used to diagnose hypoglycemia, and an additional **glucose tolerance test** or a 2-hour postprandial blood glucose test may be used to rule out diabetes. (Measurement of **sensory**

nerve conduction velocities can help diagnose diabetic neuropathy.) A low serum total calcium suggests a calcium deficiency, but for an accurate assessment of the available calcium, a **serum ionized calcium** test needs to be performed. **Potassium** levels can be checked with a serum potassium test.

Blood tests can determine **serum levels of Vitamins B-1, B-6, B-12, folic acid, and Vitamins C and D.** Any values in the lower 25% of the normal range or below would indicate that supplementation would be helpful in the treatment of trigger points. Remember that even if serum levels of vitamins and minerals are normal, you may still wish to use supplements since tissue supplies will drop before the body allows serum levels in the blood to drop.

See the above section on Nutritional Problems for comments on the digestive system and vitamin and mineral sources. See the above section on Organ Dysfunction and Disease for a discussion of thyroid function tests. A hair analysis can detect high levels of toxic metals exposure and deficiencies in minerals. A naturopathic doctor can perform **blood tests for food allergies**. Stool samples will reveal if **parasites** are a problem.

APPENDIX B

What Are Trigger Points?

Muscle Anatomy & Physiology

Muscles consist of many muscle cells, or *fibers* bundled together by connective tissue. Each fiber contains numerous *myofibrils*, and most skeletal muscles contain approximately one thousand to two thousand myofibrils. Each myofibril consists of a chain of *sarcomeres* connected end-to-end. Muscular contractions take place in the sarcomere.

A *muscle spindle* is a sensory receptor found within the belly of a muscle. Muscle spindles are concentrated where a nerve enters a muscle, and around nerves inside the muscles. Each spindle is composed of three to twelve *intrafusal muscle fibers*, which detect changes in the length of a muscle. As the body's position changes, information is conveyed to the central nervous system via sensory neurons, and is processed in the brain. As needed, the *motor end plate* (a type of nerve ending) releases *acetylcholine*, a neurotransmitter that tells the *sarcoplasmic reticulum* (part of each cell) to release ionized calcium. The *extrafusal muscle fibers* then contract. When contraction of the muscle fibers are no longer needed, the nerve ending stops releasing acetylcholine and the calcium pump within the sarcoplasmic reticulum re-uptakes calcium.

Trigger Point Physiology: Contractions and Inflammation

One of the current theories about the mechanism responsible for the formation of trigger points is the "Integrated Trigger Point Hypothesis." If a trauma occurs or there is a large increase in the motor end plate's release of acetylcholine, an excessive amount of calcium can be released by the sarcoplasmic reticulum. This causes a maximal contracture of a segment of muscle, leading to a maximal demand for energy and impairment of local circulation. If circulation is impaired, the calcium pump doesn't get the fuel and oxygen it needs to pump calcium back into the sarcoplasmic reticulum, so the muscle fiber stays contracted. Sensitizing substances are released, causing pain and stimulation of the autonomic nervous system, resulting in a positive feedback system with the motor nerve terminal releasing excessive acetylcholine...and so the sarcomere stays contracted.

Another current theory is the "Muscle Spindle" hypothesis, which proposes that the main cause of a trigger point is an inflamed muscle spindle (Partanen, Ojala, and Arokoski, 2010). Pain receptors activate skeletofusimotor units during sustained overload of muscles via a spinal reflex pathway which connect to the muscle spindles. As pain continues, sustained contraction and fatigue drive the skeletofusimotor units to exhaustion, and cause rigor (silent spasm) of the extrafusal muscle fibers, forming the "taut band" we feel as trigger points. Because the muscle spindle itself has a poor blood supply, the contraction and inflammatory metabolites released will be concentrated inside the spindle and lead to sustained inflammation.

A ground-breaking 2008 study (Shah et al.) was able to measure eleven elevated biochemicals in and surrounding active trigger points, including inflammatory mediators, neuropeptides, catecholamines, and cytokines (primarily sensitizing substances and immune system biochemicals). In addition, the pH of the samples was strongly acidic compared to other areas of the body. A 1996 study by Issbener, Reeh, and Steen found that a localized acidic pH lowers the pain threshold sensitivity level of sensory receptors (part of the nervous system), even without acute damage to the muscle. This means the more acidic your pH level in a given area, the more easily you will experience pain compared to someone else. Further studies are needed to discover whether body-wide elevations in pH acidity and the substances mentioned above predispose people to develop trigger points.

More studies are needed to determine the exact mechanisms of trigger point formation and physiology.

Central Sensitization, Trigger Points, and Chronic Pain

The *autonomic nervous system* controls the release of acetylcholine, along with involuntary functions of blood vessels and glands. Anxiety and nervous tension increase autonomic nervous system activity, which commonly aggravates trigger points and their associated symptoms.

The *central nervous system* includes the brain and spinal cord, and its function is to integrate and coordinate all activities and responses of the body. The purpose of the *acute* stress responses of our bodies is to protect us by telling us to pull away from a hot stove burner, flee from a dangerous situation, or rest an injured body part due to pain. But when emotional or physical stress is prolonged, even just for days, there is a maladaptive response: damage to the central nervous system, particularly to the sympathetic nervous system and the hypothalamus-pituitary-adrenal (HPA) systems. This is called *central nervous system sensitization.*

Pain causes certain types of nerve receptors in muscles to relay information to *neurons* located within part of the gray matter of the spinal cord and the brain stem. Pain is amplified there and then is relayed to other muscles, thereby expanding the region of pain beyond the initially affected area. Persistent pain leads to long-term or possibly permanent changes in these neurons, which affect adjacent neurons through *neurotransmitters.*

Various substances are released: *histamine* (a compound that causes dilation and permeability of blood vessels), *serotonin* (a neurotransmitter that constricts blood vessels), *bradykinin* (a hormone that dilates peripheral blood vessels and increases small blood vessel permeability), and *substance P* (a compound involved in the regulation of the pain threshold). These substances stimulate the nervous system to release even more acetylcholine locally, adding to the perpetuation of trigger points.

Central sensitization may cause the part of the nervous system that would normally counteract pain to malfunction and fail to do its job. As a result, pain can both be more easily triggered by lower levels of physical and emotional stressors, and also be more intense and last longer. Prolonged pain caused by central nervous system sensitization can lead to emotional and physical stress. Conversely, prolonged exposure to both emotional and physical stressors can lead to central nervous system sensitization and subsequently cause pain. Just the central nervous system maladaptive changes alone can be self-perpetuating and cause pain, even without the presence of either the original or any additional stressors, creating a vicious cycle of pain and trigger point formation.

Once the central nervous system is involved, because of central sensitization, even if the original perpetuating factor causing trigger points are resolved, trigger points can continue being formed and reactivated. So the longer pain goes untreated, the greater the number of neurons that get involved and the more muscles they affect, causing pain in new areas, in turn causing more neurons to get involved...the bigger the problem becomes, leading to the likelihood that pain will become chronic. The problem gets more complex, more painful, more debilitating, more frustrating, and more time-consuming and expensive to treat. The longer you wait, the less likely you are to get complete relief, and the more likely it is that your trigger points will be reactivated chronically and periodically. The sooner pain is treated, including addressing the initiating stressors and perpetuating factors, the less likely it will become a permanent problem with widespread muscle involvement and central nervous system changes.

How Will You Know if You Have Trigger Points?

The two most important characteristics of trigger points that you will notice are tender knots or tight bands in the muscles, and referred pain. You may also notice weakness, lack of range-of-motion, or other symptoms you would not normally associate with muscular problems.

Tenderness, "Knots," and Tight Bands in the Muscle

When pressed, trigger points are usually very tender. This is because the sustained contraction of the myofibril leads to the release of sensitizing neurotransmitters via a cascade effect: the sustained contraction elevates metabolites such as potassium ions and lactic acid, which leads to the elevated levels of inflammatory agents such as bradykinin and histamine, which activates pain nerve fibers, which leads to the excretion of pain transmitters, such as substance P.

Pain intensity levels can vary depending on the amount of stress placed on the muscles. The intensity of pain can also vary in response to flare-ups of any of the perpetuating factors addressed in Appendix A, and the presence of central sensitization (see above). The areas at the ends of the muscle fibers also become tender, either at the bone or where the muscle attaches to a tendon.

Healthy muscles usually do not contain knots or tight bands, are not tender to pressure, and, when not in use, feel soft and pliable to the touch, not like the hard and dense muscles found in people with chronic pain. People often tell me their muscles feel hard and dense because they work out and do strengthening exercises, but healthy muscles feel soft and pliable when not being used, even if you work out. Muscles with trigger points may also be relaxed, so don't assume you do not have trigger points just because the muscle is *not* hard and dense.

Referred Pain

Trigger points may refer pain both in the area in which the trigger point is located, and/or to other areas of the body. These are called *referral patterns.* About half of commonly found trigger points are not located within their area of referred pain. The most common referral patterns have been well documented and diagramed, and are found in the muscle chapters in section III of this book.

Unless you know where to search for trigger points, and you only work on the areas where you feel pain, you probably won't get relief. For example, trigger points in the iliopsoas muscle (deep in your abdomen) can cause pain in your lumbar area. If you don't check the iliopsoas muscle for trigger points, and only work on the quadratus lumborum muscle in the lumbar area, you will not get relief.

There are approximately four hundred muscles in the human body, but a few muscles may or may not be present in some people. Any muscle can develop trigger points, potentially causing referred pain and other symptoms. There are also individual variations in fiber or tendon arrangement, so trigger points may be located in different places for different people.

Weakness and Muscle Fatigue

Trigger points can cause weakness and loss of coordination, along with an inability to use the muscle. Many people take this as a sign that they need to strengthen the weak muscles, but you can't condition (strengthen) a muscle that contains trigger points -- these muscle fibers are not available for use because they are already contracted. If trigger points aren't inactivated first, strengthening (*conditioning*) exercises will likely encourage the surrounding muscles to do the work instead of the muscle containing the trigger point, further weakening and deconditioning the muscle containing trigger points.

Muscles containing trigger points are fatigued more easily and don't return to a relaxed state as quickly when you stop using the muscle. Trigger points may cause other muscles to tighten up and become weak and fatigued in the areas where you experience the referred pain, and also cause a generalized tightening of an area as a response to pain.

Other Symptoms

Trigger points can cause symptoms that most people would not normally associate with muscular problems. For example, trigger points in the abdominal muscles can cause urinary frequency and bladder spasms, bed-wetting, chronic diarrhea, frequent belching and gas, nausea, loss of appetite, heartburn, food intolerance, painful menses, projectile vomiting, testicular pain, and pain that feels like it is in an organ, in addition to causing referred pain in the abdominal, mid-back, and lumbar areas.

Trigger points may also cause stiff joints, generalized weakness or fatigue, twitching, trembling, and areas of numbness or other odd sensations. It probably wouldn't occur to you (or your health care provider) that these symptoms could be caused by a trigger point in a muscle.

Sensitization of the Opposite Side of the Body

For any long-term pain, it's not unusual for both sides of the body to eventually be affected; for example, if the right lumbar area is painful, there may be tender points in the left lumbar area. Often the opposite side is actually *more* tender with pressure. This is because whatever is affecting one side is likely affecting the other: poor body mechanics, poor footwear, overuse injuries, chronic degenerative or inflammatory conditions, chronic disease, or central sensitization. For that reason, I almost always treat both sides on patients, and I recommend that you do self-treatments on both sides. You may find that you have trigger points only on one side for any given muscle, but always check both sides before making that assumption.

Active Trigger Points vs. Latent Trigger Points

If a trigger point is *active*, it will refer pain or other sensations and limit range of motion. If a trigger point is *latent*, it may cause a decreased range of motion and weakness, but not pain. The more frequent and intense your pain, the greater the number of active trigger points you likely have.

Trigger points that start with some impact to the muscle, such as an injury, are usually active initially. Poor posture or poor body mechanics, repetitive use, a nerve root irritation, or any of the other perpetuating factors addressed in Appendix A can also form active trigger points. Latent trigger points can develop gradually without being active first, and you don't even know they are there. Most people have at least some latent trigger points, which can easily be converted to active trigger points.

Active trigger points may at some point stop referring pain and become latent. However, these latent trigger points can easily become active again, which may lead you to believe you're experiencing a new problem when in fact an old problem—perhaps even something you've forgotten about—is being reaggravated. Any of the perpetuating factors discussed in Appendix A can activate previously latent trigger points and make you more prone to developing new trigger points initiated by impacts to muscles.

What Initiates and Perpetuates Trigger Points?

Trigger points may form after a sudden trauma or injury, or they may develop gradually. Common initiating and perpetuating factors are mechanical stresses, injuries, nutritional problems, emotional factors, sleep problems, acute or chronic infections, organ dysfunction and disease, and other medical conditions.

You will have more control over some perpetuating factors than others. Addressing any pertinent perpetuating factors is so important that you may obtain either a great amount or complete relief from pain without any additional treatment. If you don't eliminate perpetuating factors to the extent possible, you may not get more than temporary relief from self-help pressure techniques or practitioners' treatments. Hopefully, you will learn enough about the perpetuating factors in Appendix A that at least if you choose not to resolve them, you are making an informed choice about whether the relief of pain is more important to you than continuing to do things that make you feel worse.

You cannot realistically make all of the changes in the muscle chapters and Appendix A all at once, but make a list of the perpetuating factors that might apply to you. Prioritize and work on resolving those you think might be most important.

Pain Relief with Trigger Point Self Help, DeLaune, Valerie LAc

Flashdrive format (2004, revised 2012, 2017). A multimedia book-on-Flashdrive for pain relief, appropriate for both practitioners and the lay public. It contains information on the causes and locations of trigger points for the entire body, along with hundreds of color photos with overlays of common pain referral patterns, and 144 video clips of self-help techniques for applying pressure to trigger points and performing stretches. A search feature allows you to search for your related medical conditions. Because the book navigates in your web browser, it is easy to locate the source of your pain, and move from one relevant chapter to the next.

It contains introductory chapters on the physiology and characteristics of trigger points, and a comprehensive chapter on all of the perpetuating factors that can cause and keep trigger points activated, along with solutions. Perpetuating factors include poor ergonomics and poorly-designed furniture, clothing problems, inadequate nutrition, inadequate water, improper diet, injuries, spinal and skeletal factors, sleep problems, emotional factors, allergies, hormonal imbalances, organ dysfunction or disease, and acute or chronic viral, bacterial, or parasitic infections. For more information on how to purchase this book, and for additional resources, go to http://triggerpointrelief.com/

Other Titles by Valerie DeLaune, LAc

Trigger Point Therapy Workbook for Upper Back and Neck Pain (2nd ed., 2013) Anchorage: Institute of Trigger Point Studies (e-pub, Print-on-Demand)

Trigger Point Therapy Workbook for Shoulder Pain including Frozen Shoulder (2nd ed., 2013) Anchorage: Institute of Trigger Point Studies (e-pub, Print-on-Demand)

Trigger Point Therapy Workbook for Lower Back and Gluteal Pain (2nd ed., 2013) Anchorage: Institute of Trigger Point Studies (e-pub, Print-on-Demand)

Trigger Point Therapy Workbook for Chest and Abdominal Pain (2013) Anchorage: Institute of Trigger Point Studies (e-pub)

Trigger Point Therapy Workbook for Headaches & Migraines including TMJ Pain (2013) Anchorage: Institute of Trigger Point Studies (e-pub)

Trigger Point Therapy Workbook for Lower Arm Pain including Elbow, Wrist, Hand & Finger Pain (2013) Anchorage: Institute of Trigger Point Studies (e-pub)

Trigger Point Therapy Workbook for Knee, Leg, Ankle, and Foot Pain (2018) Anchorage: Institute of Trigger Point Studies (e-pub, Print-on-Demand)

For more information on how to purchase these books, and for additional resources, go to http://triggerpointrelief.com/

"Like" the *author* on Facebook at Facebook.com: Valerie-DeLaune

"Like" the *Institute of Trigger Point Studies* on Facebook at Facebook.com: Institute-of-Trigger-Point-Studies

www.ingramcontent.com/pod-product-compliance
Lightning Source LLC
Chambersburg PA
CBHW080252030426
42334CB00023BA/2783